THE MALIGNANT PROSPECTORS

UNLOCKING THE TRUTH BEHIND
LIVING A HEALTHY CANCER-FREE LIFE
WITHOUT GMOS

Elliot Steinberg

Cover design by JuLee Brand / designchik.net

The Malignant Prospectors / Elliot Steinberg—1st ed.

Available in Paperback, Kindle, and eBook formats.
Paperback ISBN: 978-0-578-87728-0

Table of Contents

Dedication vii

Acknowledgments ix

Introduction - Catherine's Story 1

Chapter One – You Are What You Don't Eat 7

    Big Agriculture Goes High-tech 10

    Glyphosate and the Risk of Cancer 15

    Government and Commercial Testing for Pesticides 19

    Arguments Against Using GMO and Glyphosate 22

    Summary 24

Chapter Two – The Truth About Organic Food 27

    The History of Organic Food Production 27

    Definitions, Differences, and Qualifications 31

    Labeling Genetically Modified Organisms and Organic
    Products 38

    What to Look for When You Buy Organic 40

    The Dirty Dozen 41

    The Clean 15 41

    The Cost of Buying Organic 41

    Where to Shop for Organic Food 42

    Summary – Why Should You Eat Organic? 43

Chapter Three – Genetically Modified Organisms 45

    How It All Started 46

How Genetically Modified Organisms Have Evolved Over Time.. 49

Crops 50

Animals.. 52

Insects 53

The Contested Issue of GMOs 53

Claims Against GMOs 56

The Top 20 GMO Foods and Ingredients to Avoid........... 56

Summary 61

Chapter Four – GMOs, Legislation, and the Business of Cancer 63

Genetically Modifying Organisms........................... 65

The Legislation 67

Current Right to Know Activity by State 74

The Business of Cancer... 75

Government Farm Subsidies..................................... 76

The History of Farm Subsidies 77

Summary 82

Chapter Five – Regulation and the Cause for GMO Food Labeling 85

Where Labeling Stands Today.................................. 86

CRISPR-Cas9 Technology Emerges 90

What You Can Expect to See on Labeling 92

The Quiz 93

Summary 95

Chapter Six – Reducing the Burden of Cancer.................97

The Diet Connection 98

At the Center of the Debate 100

The Secrets to Buying Non-GMO..................................... 105

Summary 106

Chapter Seven – Conclusions.. 109

Roundup Ready® Gets into the Market.............................111

Organic Food Enters the Market 114

GMOs and the Threat of Cancer.. 118

References 123

About the Author 131

Dedicated to my beloved mother
Catherine Steinberg

ACKNOWLEDGMENTS

This book was made possible by
JuLee Brand of W. Brand Publishing

Catherine's Story

"I'm cold. Will you hand me a blanket?"

"Sure, Mom. Do you need anything else?

"No. I'm just going to rest for a while before dinner. I don't know why, though. I really don't feel like eating."

My mother, Catherine, was diagnosed with ovarian cancer when she was only sixty-six years old. Far too soon for a woman who still had so much of life to live.

It all started when she began complaining of abdominal pain. By the time she went in to see the doctor, we knew things weren't good when doctor sat us down and said I have very bad news to tell you. She'd need months of chemo and radiation therapy even after surgery to remove a huge mass from her ovaries and all the adjacent tissue. By the time the doctors went in, the cancer had already metastasized to her spine, lungs, and other organs: My mother was suffering from stage four ovarian cancer.

After she was diagnosed, they tried everything to ameliorate her pain until her health deteriorated to the point where doctors discussed amputating her leg due to blood clots. My mom wasn't having any of it though she said, "No matter how long I have to live, I won't let them take all my limbs" By the time she passed, she was on seventeen different pain medications and all of them at almost the highest dose possible. Mom was in so much pain, there was nothing more the doctors could do for her because the cancer had already spread so far so quickly. Early detection might have saved her, but sadly, that didn't happen.

Genetically speaking, there was no reason on earth why my mom should have been stricken with cancer at such a young age. No one in our family has ever had any form cancer at all. So for us, the genetic angle was completely ruled out. That's when it all started to point to her diet. After eliminating all of the other crazy risk factors we have today, her cancer pointed to her food. Toward the end, my mom's diet consisted of mainly fruits, berries, and the occasional bowl of oatmeal in the morning. She never ate meat, opting instead to eat fish. She was a pescatarian, but keeping in mind the direct relationship to mercury in fish, it probably wasn't the best thing for her either. That's when I first learned that farm-raised fish is loaded with GMOs to sterilize them.

Despite her diagnosis, none of us in the family were particularly aware of the underlying relationship between GMOs and cancer yet. Mom always thought that despite her cancer battle, she was relatively healthy for someone her age, and she did the best she could. Her one fallibility was perhaps the occasional microwave popcorn. She loved it and ate two or three bags a week. Of course, we didn't know about the relationship between microwave popcorn and cancer either. The bag when heated releases toxins which are absorbed by the popcorn which cause cancer too.

Mom's battle went on for nearly six years. When things got bad, we commuted to the cancer facility almost daily, but in the end, she ended up living there full time. Then when the cancer had spread to her lungs and whole body it was all over.

My mom's death struck a chord with me, I began searching for answers about how a vibrant, sixty-six-year-old woman could go so fast. I think everyone needs to be aware of what they're eating and what is really being done to our food? Food producers shouldn't be fooling around and manipulating what we consume to the degree that they currently are. That doesn't seem fair to me, but that's what the problem really is and what this book is all about.

I have three reasons for writing this book.

To provide the reader with the necessary knowledge and foresight, as to which products on the market today contain GMO's and cause cancer. Second, to decrease and perhaps even eliminate your exposure to the ubiquitous risks of cancer. Third, to help those that are currently struggling with cancer make safe choices regarding their health, by being able to know which foods may exacerbate their current condition, and pose an increase health risk.

This book is divided into seven chapters. In "You Are What You Don't Eat," I describe what happens to the food we eat when it meets high-tech science. The result isn't always pretty. The chief offender is glyphosate—a non-selective herbicide, originally designed to kill unwanted plants and insects. As with many other "good ideas," the resulting *Frankenfood*, washed in pesticides, often runs amok, permeating every aspect of our lives and causing cancer.

Chapter two, "The Truth About Organic Food" puts small farmers and big agriculture toe-to-toe and under a microscope to explain the differences between traditional commercial food and organic crop production. Do you know the difference? Can you spot the discrepancies between a bag of organic carrots from the "bargains?" I also introduce the controversy of product labeling; specifically, as it pertains to fruit, vegetables, grains, nuts, and seeds.

The third chapter, "Genetically Modified Organisms," addresses fluorescent pigs, glow-in-the-dark salmon, and goats' milk that winds up in bullet-proof vests. I put GMOs on center stage. What happens to regular food when its DNA gets tweaked by scientists and big agricultural companies? You'll also learn why GMOs and their labeling has become such a controversy.

In the fourth chapter, "GMOs, Legislation and the Business of Cancer," I bring you up to speed with the current information about genetically modified organisms, or GMOs. What are they? Where do they hide? What is the government doing, or not doing rather to legislate them and reduce the risk to the consumer? Hold onto your hat, because you're in for an adventure. What you learn may not always be comforting, but as taxpaying citizens, it's important to know where your money is going and who controls the health-related purse strings. I also set the stage so we can intelligently discuss what's happening to farmers, large-scale food production, and the laws that govern them.

In chapter five, "Regulation and the Cause for GMO Labeling" addresses GMO food labeling. Similar to the nutrition labeling that started in 1965, informing consumers about the amount of fat, protein, and carbohydrates in products, GMO packaging is designed to educate and guide consumers through their purchases; *if* they can figure out how to interpret them. Most people can't. The crazy maze of government control, together with lobbying and big agriculture sets the stage for an action thriller that puts most Hollywood blockbusters to shame.

Next, chapter six addresses "Reducing the Burden of Cancer," and I'll share some of what I've learned since my mother's passing, including the clear links between GMOs and cancer.

I'll also talk about the secrets of how to identify which non-Organic products are GMO free and which are loaded with GMO's, basically how to avoid "The Malignant Prospectors"

In the final chapter, "Conclusions," I sum up my findings, facts, and statistics. Sort of a primer for people new to genetically modified organisms.

I have to warn you, this isn't exactly light reading that will help you nod off to sleep at night. This is serious stuff that could mean the difference between life or death for many people. If you take your health seriously, then I know you will benefit tremendously and learn a lot about the relationship between what you eat and cancer.

CHAPTER ONE

You Are What You *Don't* Eat

T he Egyptian goddess Sekhmet was known as the "Lady of Pestilence" and was prone to dispensing justice over anyone who angered her. Part voluptuous Jezebel and part lioness, she was perhaps, the first example on record of mankind cross-breeding entities to fit its needs; in this case, a goddess who could rain plagues down on her enemies.

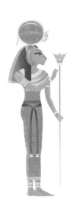

It wasn't until thousands of years later that Charles Darwin demonstrated a revolutionary concept of genetics by successfully influencing DNA in organisms. He called it "artificial selection" across similar species. By selectively breeding between two types of animals, Darwin found he could extract desired traits from one and introduce them into another resulting in new and "better" offspring.

Fast forward to the 1990s, when genetically modified foods have been approved for use in more than seventy percent of all processed foods in the United States' supermarkets Everything from pizza, potato chips, cookies, ice cream, salad dressing, corn syrup, and baking powder—just to name a few—all contain ingredients from bio-engineered soybeans, corn, or canola plants.

Even though the precursors for genetically modified foods have been around forever, it wasn't until the last forty years that they came into their own. Overnight, big agricultural businesses recognized the potential for introducing traits from other plants into soy and corn. But what slipped through the cracks during the heyday of modern genetic engineering was the link between GMOs and the threat of pesticides—particularly glyphosate. Since then, genetically engineered crops have been directly responsible for industrial and chemical-intensive models of farming, resulting in harm to wildlife, people, and the environment.

The first breakthrough in GMO technology came in the United States in 1973 when Herbert Boyer and Stanley Cohen engineered the first successful genetically engineered (GE) organism. Together, they developed a way to transfer the gene that encoded antibiotic resistance from one strain of bacteria into another, resulting in antibiotic resistance in the host.

Instead of researching long-term solutions, modern-day agriculture relies on quick fixes like dousing fertilizers and pesticides on crops as an immediate solution for large-scale food production.

As the new technology suggested exciting areas in research possibilities, the media, government, and science were already concerned with the potential ramifications it might have on human health and humanity at large. They agreed to a moratorium on all genetically engineered organisms until they understood what was at stake and how to manage its benefits and threats. Recognizing the power of their discovery, members of the scientific community and government officials convened at the Asilomar Conference of 1975 in California, and agreed to debate the future of genetic engineering. The members collectively agreed that GE projects should be allowed to continue, but with certain guidelines in place. The conference marked the first—and the last—time they would all work together.

One issue the members of the Asilomar Conference failed to address was how to bolster trust and confidence in consumers. Who should consumers believe in the upcoming battles between government, major health groups such as the American Medical Association, and big business? It set the stage for our current, ongoing bickering.

It's safe to say that since its inception, there have been as many quarrels as benefits over genetically engineered organisms; in particular, food. While some opposition is attributed to religious or philosophical values, the bulk of the brawling centers around environmental and health concerns. Many believe that dinking around with organisms' DNA is tantamount to an invitation for cancer. There's plenty of new evidence to suggest they could be right.

America's population has more than doubled since the postwar days of the early 1950s. Yet the total amount of arable land used to raise crops and feed that population has increased by less than ten percent. As a result, there's been pressure to provide more low-cost food on less land that is slowly becoming stripped of nutrients from the soil. Instead of researching long-term solutions, modern-day agriculture relies on quick fixes— such as dousing crops with fertilizers and pesticides— as an immediate solution for large-scale food production. Some of these, including the infamous pesticide DDT, are still around even after being banned as a toxic substance in 1972.

The wallop from toxic pesticides has increased exponentially over the past thirty years. At the same time, efforts to understand their impact on human health has revealed strong statistical relationships between pesticide exposure with the enhanced risk of developing neurological and immune disorders as well as numerous types of cancer.

From embryos to the aged, there are virtually no demographics escaping the risk from exposure to pesticides. Nevertheless, definitive proof that exposure to pesticides causes diseases and conditions in humans is sorely lacking. Clouding the issue is the complex threat of multi-causal exposure. Most people alive today are regularly exposed to a variety of ever-changing chemicals, not just pesticides. More importantly, there are no long-term research studies on the effects of pesticides and genetically modified organisms on human beings. But it's not for a lack of trying.

Big Agriculture Goes High-tech

Ninety percent of foods grown in the U.S. use GMO techniques for raising corn, soybean, canola, sugar beet, alfalfa, cotton, potatoes, papaya, summer squash, and a few varieties of apples. Americans have dumped more than 1.8 million tons of glyphosate on crops since its introduction in 1974. Worldwide, more than 9.4 million tons of the chemical has been sprayed on fields; enough to spray half a pound of Roundup® on every cultivated acre of land in the world. Glyphosate use has risen fifteen-fold since Roundup Ready® GMO crops were first introduced.

At the center of the controversy over GMO crops is Bt corn: a genetically modified strain grown to produce the insecticide Bt toxin[1]. Using the Bt toxin, crops can withstand insects and pests, reducing the need for pesticides. The Bt gene comes from a naturally occurring bacteria known as *Bacillus thuringiensis* and is genetically engineered and inserted into crops such as corn, cotton, and soybeans—all of which comprise more than seventy percent of commercial crops. The Bt gene produces a specific protein that is toxic to outside threats (such as insects) giving GMO plants a natural resistance. Then along came glyphosate.

To enhance production on already tweaked GM crops, farmers and large-scale agriculture companies began spraying crops with pesticides containing glyphosates[2] to kill invading broadleaf weeds and grasses.

The most common herbicide in the world, glyphosate is found in more than 750 products sold in the U.S., including these popular brands:

- Ortho GroundClear®
- Roundup®
- RM43 Total Vegetation Control®
- Compare-N-Save Concentrate Grass and Weed Killer®

---

1 GMO Science - Are all forms of Bt toxin safe? - https://www.gmoscience.org/is-bt-toxin-safe/

2 United State Environmental Protection Agency: Glyphosate - https://www.epa.gov/ingredients-used-pesticide-products/glyphosate

- Dow Rodeo Herbicide®
- Ranger Pro Herbicide®

Since its inception, glyphosate products have consistently come under fire for their risk to human and animal populations. Opinions from scientists, consumers, and advocates against its use have shot through the stratosphere:

- A statement by the International Federation of Gynecology and Obstetrics (FIGO) Reproductive and Environmental Health Committee[3] noted: "We recommend that glyphosate exposure to populations should end with a full global phase-out."
- An essay in the *Journal of Epidemiology and Community Health*[4] asked, "Is it time to reassess safety standards for glyphosate-based herbicides?"
- A consensus statement published in the *Environmental Health Journal*[5] read, "Concerns over use of glyphosate-based herbicides and risks associated with exposures: a consensus statement"
- Representing the public, a comment submitted to the EPA[6] in October 2019 by Patrick Breysse, director of the National Center for Environmental Health and

---

3 Removal of glyphosate from global usage: A Statement by the FIGO (International Federation of Gynecology and Obstetrics) Committee on Reproductive and Developmental Environmental Health - https://www.figo.org/removal-glyphosate-global-usage

4 BMJ Journal: Epidemiology and Community Health: Is it time to reassess current safety standards for glyphosate-based herbicides?

5 BMC Environmental Health: Concerns over use of glyphosate-based herbicides and risks associated with exposures: a consensus statement - https://ehjournal.biomedcentral.com/articles/10.1186/s12940-016-0117-0

6 Toxicological Profile for Glyphosate - https://www.regulations.gov/document?D=EPA-HQ-OPP-2009-0361-14366

the Agency for Toxic Substances revealed that several research papers supported the cancer connection to glyphosate and that the chemical should be banned. "Numerous studies have linked its use to an increase in lymphomas," said Breysse. "It's time we stopped letting the chemical industry manipulate research to serve its own interest. U.S. citizens need to trust the Environmental Protection Agency to operate in our best interest, which means weighing evidence from neutral scientific sources not vested in the outcome."

- In 2015, the World Health Organization's International Agency for Research on Cancer (IARC) classified glyphosate as "probably carcinogenic to humans[7]" after reviewing years of published and peer-reviewed scientific studies. The team of international scientists found there was a particular association between glyphosate and Non-Hodgkin's Lymphoma.

While the IARC was making its classification, the Environmental Protection Agency was busy conducting counter-reviews of its own. The EPA's Cancer Assessment Review Committee (CARC) issued a report in September 2016 [8]concluding that glyphosate was "not likely to be carcinogenic to humans" at doses relevant to human health—whatever "relevant to human health" means. Following these findings, the EPA convened a scientific advisory panel to review the report. Members were equally divided in their assessment of the

---

7 IARC Monographs Volume 112: evaluation of five organophosphate insecticides and herbicide - https://www.iarc.fr/wp-content/uploads/2018/07/MonographVolume112-1.pdf

8 Glyphosate Issue Paper: Evaluation of Carcinogenic Potential - https://www.epa.gov/sites/production/files/2016-09/documents/glyphosate_issue_paper_evaluation_of_carcincogenic_potential.pdf

EPA's work, with some members finding that the EPA erred in how it evaluated and disseminated the results of its research.

Since glyphosate products were introduced to the market, more than 42,000 people have filed lawsuits against Monsanto Company.

The EPA's Office of Research and Development claimed that EPA's Office of Pesticide Programs had not followed proper protocols in its evaluation of glyphosate[9], yet said that the resulting evidence could be deemed to support a "likely" carcinogenic or "suggestive" evidence of carcinogenicity classification. Nevertheless, the EPA issued a draft report[10] on glyphosate in December 2017 insisting that the chemical was not likely to be carcinogenic. In April 2019, the EPA reaffirmed its position that glyphosate posed no risk to public health, even though earlier in the same month, the U.S. Agency for Toxic Substances and Disease Registry (ATSDR) reported links between glyphosate and cancer. According to the draft report from ATSDR, "Numerous studies reported risk ratios greater than one for associations between glyphosate exposure and risk of Non-Hodgkin's Lymphoma or multiple myeloma." The conflict didn't end there.

---

9 Summary of ORO comments on OPP's glyphosate cancer assessment December 14, 2015 - https://usrtk.org/wp-content/uploads/2017/03/ORDcommentsonOPPglyphosate.pdf

10 EPA Releases Draft Risk Assessments for Glyphosate - https://www.epa.gov/pesticides/epa-releases-draft-risk-assessments-glyphosate

In 2016, the World Health Organization's Joint Meeting on Pesticide Residues[11] determined that glyphosate was unlikely to pose a carcinogenic risk to humans from exposure through diet, but the finding was tarnished by concerns over conflicts of interest after it was learned that the chair and co-chair of the group also held leadership positions with the International Life Sciences Institute, a group funded in part by Monsanto and one of its lobbying organizations.

Finally, on March 28, 2017, the California Environmental Protection Agency's Office of Environmental Health Hazard Assessment (OEHHA) confirmed it would add glyphosate to California's Proposition 65 list of chemicals known to cause cancer. In a separate case, the court found that California could not require cancer warnings for products containing glyphosate. On June 12, 2018, a U.S. District Court denied the California Attorney General's request for the court to reconsider the decision. The court ruled that California could only require commercial speech that disclosed "purely factual and uncontroversial information," because, at the time, the science surrounding glyphosate carcinogenicity was not yet proven. And so, the battle wages on.

Glyphosate and the Risk of Cancer

Since glyphosate products were introduced to the market, more than 42,000 people have filed lawsuits against Monsanto Company claiming that exposure to its Roundup® herbicide caused them or their loved ones to develop Non-Hodgkin's Lymphoma (NHL) and that Monsanto covered up *known* risks.

---

11 Joint FAO/WHO Meeting On Pesticide Residues - https://www.who.int/foodsafety/jmprsummary2016.pdf

The first trial ended in a large award to the plaintiffs for liability and damages, with the jury ruling that Monsanto's weed killer was a substantial contributing factor in causing them to develop NHL. The current owner, Bayer, is appealing the ruling.

But the lawsuit that really got the public's attention was the high-profile, 2014 case of Dewayne Johnson[12] against Monsanto. Johnson was a former school groundskeeper diagnosed with terminal NHL. In August 2018, a judge ordered Monsanto to pay Johnson $289 million in damages. The award was subsequently reduced to $78 million after Monsanto appealed.

One thing that all of the lawsuits have in common is the plaintiff's claim that Roundup® was a "defective" product and Monsanto knew that glyphosate caused cancer.

Johnson's action was followed by another suit filed in the U.S. District Court in Los Angeles on Sept. 22, 2015. The plaintiff was 58-year-old Enrique Rubio, a former farmworker in California, Texas, and Oregon who labored in cucumber and onion fields as well as other vegetable crops. Some of his duties included spraying fields with Roundup® and other pesticides until he was diagnosed with bone cancer in 1995. Attorney Robin Greenwald, one of the attorneys who brought forth Rubio's case, said she expects more lawsuits to follow because Roundup® is the most widely used herbicide in the world. She said, "I believe there will be hundreds of lawsuits brought over time." She was correct.

---

12 Jurors give $289 million to a man they say got cancer from Monsanto's Roundup weed killer - https://www.cnn.com/2018/08/10/health/monsanto-johnson-trial-verdict/index.html

Finally, a lawsuit making similar claims was filed in federal court in New York by 64-year-old Judi Fitzgerald, who was diagnosed with leukemia in 2012. Fitzgerald claimed she was exposed to Roundup® in the early 1990s when she worked at a horticultural products company. Monsanto spokeswoman Charla Lord argued that the claims were without merit and that glyphosate is safe for humans when used as directed on the product labels: "Decades of experience within agriculture and regulatory reviews using the most extensive worldwide human health databases ever compiled on an agricultural product contradict the claims in the suit which will be vigorously defended."

One thing that all of the lawsuits have in common are the plaintiffs' claim that Roundup® was a "defective" product and "unreasonably dangerous" to consumers, that Monsanto knew—or *should* have known—that glyphosate caused cancer and other illnesses, and failed to properly warn consumers of the risks. Further, the lawsuits also claimed that the Environmental Protection Agency changed an initial classification for glyphosate from "possibly carcinogenic to humans" to "evidence of non-carcinogenicity in humans" after pressure from Monsanto. World Health Organization scientists cited several studies showing cancer links to glyphosate, though Monsanto has said the findings are wrong.

On Oct 6, 2017, Jeffrey Smith, Executive Director of the Institute for Responsible Technology delivered a lecture at the Truth About Cancer Conference in Orlando, Florida. During his speech, he explained:

- The very process of creating a GMO creates side effects that can promote cancer. Monsanto's Roundup Ready® corn, for example, has higher levels of putrescine and cadaverine. These are not only linked to cancer but also to allergies.

- Bt-toxin, which is manufactured by the altered DNA in every cell of genetically modified varieties of corn, cotton, and South American soy, pokes holes in cell walls. It may create "leaky gut," which is linked to cancer and numerous other diseases.

- Most GMOs are "Roundup Ready®"—designed to be sprayed with Monsanto's Roundup® herbicide. These include soy, corn, cotton, canola, sugar beets (for sugar), and alfalfa. Glyphosate, the active ingredient in Roundup®, is classified as a class 2A carcinogen by the International Agency for Research on Cancer (part of the World Health Organization). The agency says it *probably* causes cancer in humans, *does* cause cancer in animals, *does* cause mutations in DNA that can lead to cancer, and where it is heavily sprayed, cancer rates are higher.

- Roundup® is also sprayed on numerous non-GMO crops just before harvest as a desiccant (called "green burndown") to dry the crop and reduce the amount of time until harvest. Some of the affected crops sprayed with Roundup® include wheat, oats, flax, peas, lentils, dry beans, sugar cane, rye, triticale, buckwheat, millet, canola, corn, soybeans, potatoes, and sunflowers labeled non-GMO.

- Several cancer rates in the U.S. are rising in parallel with the increased use of glyphosate on GMO soy and cornfields. These include leukemia and cancers of the liver, kidney, bladder, thyroid, and breast.

- In Argentina, the rate of cancer in communities living near Roundup Ready® soybean fields has skyrocketed.

Soaring increased rates are also seen with birth defects, thyroid conditions, lupus, and respiratory problems.

- To avoid using Roundup®-coated crops, eating non-GMO food is not sufficient. It is better to choose organic, which does not allow the use of GMOs, Roundup®, or other synthetic poisons. Products labeled both Organic and Non-GMO Project Verified are even better because the latter requires tests for possible inadvertent GMO contamination.

The following are some of the health effects of glyphosate that we know of—all of which are known to increase the risk of cancer. Glyphosate:

- Damages the DNA
- Is an antibiotic
- Promotes leaky gut
- Chelates minerals, making them unavailable
- Is toxic to the mitochondria
- Interferes with key metabolic pathways
- Causes non-alcoholic fatty liver disease
- Degrades into sarcosine and formaldehyde

Government and Commercial Testing for Pesticides

One way to placate consumers and avoid future litigation, of course, is for Monsanto and other big chemical companies to admit the truth, test their products, and display the results on product labels. But until big business gets out of bed with the government, it simply won't happen. There is no impetus to discover and label toxic products when they represent millions of dollars in revenue for BigAg companies, lobbyists, and the government. The United States Department of Agriculture data from 2016 showed detectable pesticide levels in eighty-five percent of more than 10,000 foods sampled—everything from mushrooms to grapes and green beans. At the same time, the government claims there are little to no health risks[13], but with so much money and influence on the line, it's not likely to turn a blind eye and admit the truth.

In March 2017, a federal court judge unsealed internal Monsanto documents that raised new questions about its influence on the EPA process and the research regulators it depends on. The documents suggested that Monsanto's long-standing claims about the safety of glyphosate and Roundup® do not necessarily rely on sound practices as the company asserts, but instead on efforts to manipulate the science.

The FDA actually began limited testing for pesticides in early 2016, but the effort was fraught with controversy and internal difficulties, so the program was suspended in September 2016. Internal FDA documents obtained by the advocacy group, "U.S. Right to Know" showed that the FDA had planned to start testing more than 300 samples of corn syrup for glyphosate beginning in April 2017, but it killed the project before it got started.

The USDA data from 2016 shows detectable pesticide levels in eighty-five percent of more than 10,000 foods sampled. At the same time, the government claims there are little to no health risks.

---

13 Chemicals on our food: When "safe" may not really be safe - https://www.ehn.org/when-safe-may-not-really-be-safe-2621578745.html

Before the suspension, one FDA chemist found alarming levels of glyphosate in samples of domestic honey—levels that were technically illegal because there had never been allowable levels established for honey by the EPA. Independent testing by the consumer group "Food Democracy Now" found high levels of glyphosate in Cheerios breakfast cereal, oatmeal cookies, Ritz crackers, and other popular brands of snack foods.

In October 2018, the FDA issued its first-ever report showing the results of glyphosate residue in food testing[14]. According to FDA data, no glyphosate residues were found in milk or eggs, but residues were found in more than sixty-three percent of corn samples and sixty-seven percent of soybean samples.

Finally, *Consumer Reports* magazine, which is highly critical of GMOs, included a comment by Robert Gould, president of the board of Physicians for Social Responsibility, in a 2015 commentary[15]: "The contention that GMOs pose no risks to human health can't be supported by studies that have measured a time frame that is too short to determine the effects of exposure over a lifetime."

Does all this sound familiar? If you're one of the thousands of people who got hooked on cigarettes by big tobacco back in the 1950s and 1960s, you know that big business and the government can't be trusted to tell consumers the truth; the very people who keep them in business and make them rich. After years of litigation and lower consumer sales, big

---

14 FDA Tests Confirm Oatmeal, Baby Foods Contain Residues of Monsanto Weed Killer - https://www.huffpost.com/entry/fda-tests-confirm-oatmeal_b_12252824

15 GMO foods: What you need to know - https://www.consumerreports.org/cro/magazine/2015/02/gmo-foods-what-you-need-to-know/index.htm

tobacco companies finally folded and were forced to start labeling their products.

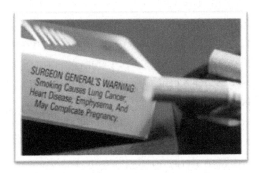

Arguments Against Using GMO and Glyphosate

Although hotly contested, current research suggests that glyphosate has been found to increase the risk of blood cancer, NHL, and the risk of related cancer, and multiple myeloma. Multiple myeloma was recently classified as a sub-type of NHL, even though the two were once considered distinct diseases.

In a report released in late July 2015, the world's leading cancer experts at the International Agency for Research on Cancer shed new light on the cancer-causing properties of glyphosate. The report[16] took an in-depth look at the latest research and concluded that glyphosate is definitely carcinogenic to animals in laboratory studies, and that human exposure is linked to a higher risk of developing blood cancers such as NHL.

---

16 World Health Organization: Some Organophosphate Insecticides and Herbicides - https://publications.iarc.fr/549

Misinformation, shady marketing, and biased lawmaking
have ensued—not to mention the damage
that is yet to be seen as an entire generation
grows up on Frankenfoods.

The authors of a University of Washington report[17] analyzed all published studies on the impact of glyphosate on humans. Co-author and doctoral student Rachel Shaffer said in a statement: "This research provides the most up-to-date analysis of glyphosate and its link with NHL, incorporating a 2018 study of more than 54,000 people who work as licensed pesticide applicators."

Concentrating on data relating to people with the "highest exposure" to the herbicide, researchers concluded that a "compelling link" exists between glyphosate exposure and a greater risk of developing NHL. Senior author Lianne Sheppard, a professor in biostatistics and environmental and occupational health sciences said she was "convinced" of the carcinogenic properties of the chemical. Predictably, in an opposing statement, Bayer called the new analysis a "statistical manipulation" with "serious methodological flaws," adding that it "provides no scientifically valid evidence that contradicts the conclusions of the extensive body of science demonstrating that glyphosate-based herbicides are not carcinogenic."

Even more confounding are the lobbying efforts behind GMOs that feed untold amounts of cash and have a vested interest in protecting their clients' practices. As a result,

17 UW study: Exposure to chemical in Roundup increases risk for cancer - https://www.washington.edu/news/2019/02/13/uw-study-exposure-to-chemical-in-roundup-increases-risk-for-cancer/

misinformation, shady marketing, and biased lawmaking have ensued, leading to health problems and lawsuits—not to mention the damage that is yet to be seen as an entire generation grows up on *Frankenfood.*

Summary

These days, it's relatively easy to hug the perimeter of the grocery store to shop for organic fruits and vegetables, and avoid boxed carcinogens that lie deep within the store's center aisles. Unfortunately, even if you gather your own real ingredients in the produce section where food looks like "food," choosing non-GMO products can be precarious and sometimes dangerous. We have GMOs and their connection to cancer to thank for that.

The World Health Organization tells us that popular herbicides and pesticides are "probably carcinogenic," citing links between glyphosate and animal tumors as well as genetic damage in humans after glyphosate exposure[18].

But here's where the rubber meets the road. Our circulating DNA is *already* afflicted. Our digestive systems are damaged from years of eating so-called "whole foods" that are "low-fat" and "gluten-free." Our children—even those who are just beginning their lives in utero, are already exposed to hundreds of toxins, with the threat of cancer around every turn.

Consumer advocates with "no dog in the race" suggest compelling reasons why we shouldn't trust the government and big business. They're all in it for the money.

---

18 World Health Organization: Evaluation of five organophosphate insecticides and herbicides - https://www.iarc.fr/wp-content/uploads/2018/07/MonographVolume112-1.pdf

German scientists discovered in 2014[19] that years of toxic substances chipping away at our internal systems lead to chronic illness and premature death. People with chronic illness were found to have "significantly higher" herbicide residue in their urine than healthy individuals. Nevertheless, the current research on the health risks of GMOs still remains inconclusive. In other words, researchers cannot confirm whether or not GMOs increase cancer risks, and as long as there is so much money at stake, they never will.

Knowing who to trust and what to believe is an ongoing, personal battle. Major health groups—including the American Medical Association and World Health Organization—that we've come to respect and turn to for valid information have concluded from their research of independent groups worldwide that genetically modified foods are safe for consumers; that they are free of threats to organ health, mutations, pregnancy, and offspring. At the same time, however, consumer advocates have presented startling information to the contrary. Consumer advocates with "no dogs in the race" suggest compelling reasons why we shouldn't trust the government and big business. They're all in it for the money.

———————————

Although scientists have been able to manipulate data indicating that GMOs are not toxic to the animals that eat them, they've failed to support long-term studies in humans. Despite the heavy and increasing use of GMOs—and the subsequent pervasive use of chemicals that follows—long-term evaluations

———————————

19 Journal of Environmental & Analytical Toxicology: Detection of Glyphosate Residues in Animals and Humans - https://www.hilarispublisher.com/open-access/detection-of-glyphosate-residues-in-animals-and-humans-2161-0525.1000210.pdf

ensuring human safety are nowhere to be found. Why? Because government and big business like things exactly the way they are, making money hand over fist with little or no concern over the health of consumers. . .in the way big tobacco felt back in the 1950s.

The tide won't begin to turn until consumers take more responsibility. That means buying organic and non-GMO products, sharing current information with their friends, colleagues, and neighbors, and increasing their voices through larger-scale activism. At the most basic level, consumers have a responsibility to speak with their wallets, to be selective about what they buy, and what they put into their bodies. It's the only way farmers, government, and big business will listen.

CHAPTER TWO

The Truth About Organic Food

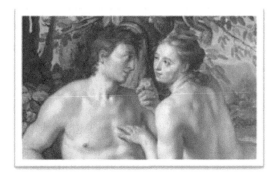

F ive minutes after Adam offered Eve an apple he bought from The Garden of Eden Whole Foods Market, she was all over him: "Adam, is this apple organic? Does it contain GMOs? What about pesticides?" The rest is history.

The History of Organic Food Production

By the late 1940s, the role of pesticides began impacting American agriculture in a big way. Countries decimated from the war were desperate to quickly boost food production, so they introduced the insecticide DDT to eliminate disease-carrying insects. At the same time, companies such as I.G. Farben—the producer of the infamous poison "Zyklon B" used in gas chambers at concentration camps—was looking for new markets and ways to resuscitate its tarnished image. Eventually, Farben broke up into a number of smaller companies. Two of them were B.A.SF and Bayer, some of the largest agricultural chemical companies today. Bayer later purchased a third player, Monsanto.

Farmers noticed that by spraying synthetic insecticides and fertilizers on their crops, they could significantly boost production. Spraying became an integral part of "modern-day" farming. Heeding America's reputation for supersizing, farmers depending on government subsidies were pressured by Secretary of Agriculture Earl Butz to "Get big or get out."

At the same time, a completely different approach to feeding America was taking root. The American version of *An Agricultural Testament*[20] was published in 1943 and sparked the interest of J.I. Rodale, founder of the pioneering research organization, the Soil and Health Foundation, now called the Rodale Institute.

Founders were concerned that consumers were being duped by large scale growers trying to muscle their way into the popularity of organic food sales.

---

20 By Sir Albert Howard. London, New York and Toronto: Oxford University Press, 1940.

In 1962, conservationist Rachel Carson published *Silent Spring*[21], one of the first books warning about the negative relationship between agricultural pesticides and damage to the environment. In response, the long-haired, tie-dyed, Birkenstock-wearing counter-culture movement of the 1960s and 1970s began to embrace the so-called "back to the land" movement that preached eating whole foods, twigs, berries, and smoking pot that was grown without commercial fertilizers and pesticides. But the movement was much more than just shunning commercial pesticides. It started a revolution that preached environmental stewardship, family health, and introduced the concept of "buying local" directly from organic farmers.

As the popularity of organic food slowly seeped into large chain grocery stores, the organic certification evolution took hold. The founders were concerned that consumers were being duped by large-scale growers trying to muscle their ways into the popularity of organic food sales. Their solution was the first set of standards identifying organic food packaging.

In 1973, Oregon became the first state to pass a law regulating organic food production. That was followed by Congress passing the Organic Foods Production Act[22] in 1990. Even with established law, however, there was constant bickering over what the act entailed and how it should be enforced. After several failed attempts, a final rule establishing the U.S. Department of Agriculture (USDA) organic standards went into effect in February, 2001.

---

21 Rachel Carson. Houghton Mifflin Company; Anniversary edition (October 22, 2002)

22 Organic Foods Production Act of 1990 - https://www.ams.usda.gov/sites/default/files/media/Organic%20Foods%20Production%20Act%20of%201990%20(OFPA).pdf

Instantly, large-scale commercial farmers began cutting corners, "misinterpreting," or shall we say, "bending the law" to their benefit as they tried to take advantage of lax USDA enforcement. "It's a failure in the system," says Cornucopia Institute co-founder Mark Kastel. "Now you have to look for this label *and* do your homework." One example is the definition of "organic" when applied to raising cows for beef and milk production. The law states that in order to call its products organic, farmers must ensure that cows have free access to pasture at least 120 days per year. The founding fathers of the law envisioned seas of bovine leisurely grazing on acres of lush, green grass. The reality was many commercial food producers ended up stuffing as many as a dozen cows into cramped, grass-lined stalls for the minimum amount of time in order to meet USDA-mandated standards.

As the organic food production industry matures, organic farmers and food producers face stiff competition from large companies who primarily produce conventional food, yet want to slither in through the back door of organic products, eschewing formal practices. The maker of Nature's Path cereal was one of the first to throw up their hands, bailing out of the Organic Trade Organization through a press release citing the association's support for controversial new memberships, such as B.A.SF, one of the world's largest producers of pesticides, and Cargill, a company that dominates the market for GMO livestock feed used in Concentrated Animal Feeding Operations (CAFOs). The *Organic Insider* newsletter[23] broke a story through an impassioned post outlining how misaligned the interests of the two companies were with the true organic mission.

---

23 *Organic Insider* - https://organicinsider.com/

Definitions, Differences, and Qualifications

In theory, organic standards used for commercially grown foods are "process-based," meaning they dictate the entire process of organic food production from its inception on the farm all the way to retail outlets. Those rules specifically dictate processes for planting, growing, raising, and handling.

Large-scale commercial farmers began cutting corners, "misinterpreting," or bending the law to their benefit.

The USDA organic label on dairy and meat products means that "the animals from which it originated were raised in living conditions that accommodated their natural behaviors, without being administered hormones or antibiotics, and while grazing on pasture grown on healthy soil. During processing, the meat or dairy product must be handled in a facility that is inspected by an organic certifier and processed without any artificial colors, preservatives, or flavors before being packaged to avoid contact with any prohibited, non-organic substances." Whew. That's a mouthful. But there's more.

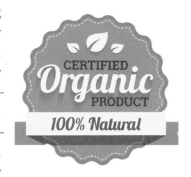

In the United States, organic crops must be grown without using synthetic pesticides, bioengineered genes (GMOs), petroleum-based, and sewage sludge-based fertilizers. Organic livestock raised for eggs and dairy products is required to have access to the outdoors and be given organic feed. They must not be given antibiotics, growth hormones, or any animal by-products. Organic food such as vegetables, fruit, eggs, milk, and meat must also be produced without synthetic pesticides, herbicides, and fertilizers. On the other hand, organic farmers may use natural pesticides if they've been approved for organic food production by the USDA.

There are several levels of organic labeling being used today in the manufacture of consumer products:

1. **One hundred percent organic:** Foods grown with exclusive, organic-certified ingredients.
2. **Organic:** At least ninety-five percent of the ingredients in these foods are organic.
3. **Made with Organic:** At least seventy percent of ingredients in these foods are made using organic farming practices.

In practice, "one hundred percent organic" can be used to label just about any product that contains all organic ingredients (excluding salt and water, which are considered natural). Most raw, unprocessed farm products are "one hundred percent organic," as well as many grains, oats, and flours. Similarly, but not exactly the same, "Organic" can be used to label any product that contains less than five percent non-organic agricultural products.

Produce can be called organic if it's certified to have grown on soil that has no prohibited substances applied for three years prior to harvest. Prohibited substances include most synthetic fertilizers and pesticides. In instances when a grower has to use a synthetic substance to achieve a specific purpose, the substance must first be approved according to criteria that examine its effects on human health and the environment.

Organically raised animals should never be given antibiotics, growth hormones, or fed animal by-products. They risk getting mad cow disease and Bovine Spongiform Encephalopathy (BSE). They can also create antibiotic-resistant strains of bacteria.

In the U.S., organic food is big business. Seventy percent of organic foods purchased include fruits and vegetables. They're pricey because approved farming practices are more expensive to follow. So, why on earth should you plunk down your hard-earned cash to eat organic when there are so many other less expensive options? It's simple: Quality.

Organic meat and milk are richer in nutrients than non-organic products. Results of a 2016 European study showed that levels of Omega-3 fatty acids were fifty percent higher in organic meat and milk than in conventionally raised versions. Organic food is also free of GMOs or genetically engineered (GE) foods whose DNA has been altered in ways that cannot occur in nature or traditional crossbreeding, most commonly to be resistant to pesticides or produce insecticides. But does eating organic mean that you're eating food free of pesticides? The short answer is *maybe*.

One of the primary benefits of eating organic is lower levels of pesticides. However, despite popular belief, organic farms do occasionally use them. The difference is they are restricted to naturally derived pesticides rather than the synthetic chemicals used on conventional farms. Natural pesticides are believed to be less toxic, however, some have also been found to represent health risks.

The U.S. market is the easiest for potentially fraudulent organic products to penetrate because the chances of getting caught are not very high

For multi-ingredient foods, the USDA organic standards prohibit organically processed foods from containing artificial preservatives, åcolors or flavors, and require their ingredients to be organic, with some minor exceptions. For example, processed organic foods may contain some approved non-agricultural ingredients, such as enzymes in yogurt, pectin in fruit jams, or baking soda in baked goods. Are you confused yet? Read on. It gets worse.

Organic product sales reached nearly $50 billion in 2017[24] and demand still vastly outstrips supply, sometimes leading to outright fraud. A 2016 *Washington Post* investigation[25] discovered that in the rush to satisfy demand, millions of pounds of soybeans and corn purchased from Turkey were sold into the U.S. market as organic, but had actually been grown using conventional farming practices. The story began with thirty-six million pounds of soybeans that sailed from Ukraine to Turkey, and finally to California. The soybeans started their journey as ordinary soybeans that were fumigated with pesticides and priced similarly to ordinary soybeans. By the time the cargo ship carrying the soybeans arrived on the West Coast, they had mysteriously been labeled "USDA

---

24 Organic Trade Association - Organic Industry Survey - https://ota.com/organic-market-overview/organic-industry-survey

25 Washington Post - *The labels said 'organic.' But these massive imports of corn and soybeans weren't.* - https://www.washingtonpost.com/business/economy/the-labels-said-organic-but-these-massive-imports-of-corn-and-soybeans-werent/2017/05/12/6d165984-2b76-11e7-a616-d7c8a68c1a66_story.html

Organic;" a switch that increased their value by more than $4 million.

When *Washington Post* contacted the original source of the soybeans, it simply admitted that "it may have been 'provided with false certification documents.'" The inquiry demonstrated how fallible the "USDA Organic" label really is, and exposed the weaknesses in the current system. The Agriculture Department said it was investigating the fraudulent organic shipments, but declined to identify any of the firms or shipments involved.

Regardless of where organics come from, the system suffers from multiple weaknesses in enforcement. First off, farmers are free to hire their own subjective inspectors. Secondly, most inspections are announced days or weeks in advance eliminating the element of surprise, and finally, testing for pesticides is the exception rather than the rule. Even though the U.S. has tripled the amount of imported soybeans and "organic" corn from other countries, the USDA has done nothing more to stop illegitimate practices.

"The U.S. market is the easiest for potentially fraudulent organic products to penetrate because the chances of getting caught here are not very high," said John Bobbe, Executive Director of the Organic Farmers Agency for Relationship Marketing, or OFARM, a farmer's cooperative. "In Europe and Canada," he continued, "Import rules for organics are much stricter."

In China, farmers have trouble following their own laws,
so how can Americans expect Chinese farmers
will follow U.S. organic rules?

When the USDA does respond to complaints about questionable imports, it's usually too late to do anything to rectify the problem. By that time, the products have already reached their customers, who are oblivious to the true nature of their purchases. Four months after the previously described shipment of Turkish soybeans reached their destination in California, more than twenty-one million pounds of the thirty-six million pound shipment had already reached the farms and mills, with the customers unaware that they hadn't bought truly organic products. And the story doesn't stop there.

China is the leading source of organic tea and ginger in the U.S., and its food exports have drawn repeated scrutiny. "In China, farmers have trouble following their own laws," said Chenglin Liu, a professor at St. Mary's University School of Law in San Antonio. "So how can Americans expect Chinese farmers will follow U.S. organic rules?" One investigation showed high levels of pesticide residue on some "organic" Chinese products. It also showed that pesticide residue tests are haphazardly applied. When Ceres, a German company, conducted tests on products from Chinese organic farms, it discovered that more than thirty-seven percent of their products contained traces of pesticide residue.

Even if companies purchase from honest, conscientious organic farmers, their products can become infected from polluted soil and water from neighboring farms or pollen floating in the wind. "After the ginger is washed, the water leaves behind pesticide residues too high to be considered organic in the United States," said Li Hongtao, a sales manager at the Laiwu Manhing Vegetables Fruits Corporation in Shandong, China. He said, "The ginger is sold as organic in some countries, but not the U.S. or Europe."

Even if companies purchase from honest, conscientious organic farmers, their products can become infected from polluted soil and water from neighboring farms or pollen floating in the wind.

There's also the issue of wide results from different testing companies. When Ceres investigated three hundred sixty of the ginger samples, they found remarkably high levels of pesticide revenue, while Ecocert, a French inspection company, reported only one percent in the samples tested. The problem is that different testing firms use different methods and standards. There's no one objective method for obtaining results. Critics claim that for a price, certifying agencies can make any farm appear to be organic. "The certifying agencies can choose who and when they test," said Mischa Popoff, a former USDA organic inspector-turned-critic. "That's why the results they can get are completely arbitrary."

According to USDA statistics from 2014 to 2016, the United States saw an increase of organic corn from 15,000 metric tons to 399,000 metric tons originating from Turkey. The rise in imports helped drop prices by more than twenty-five percent, which hurt U.S. organic farmers, many of them small operations. "There are challenges with the complex supply chain of organic grain," said one USDA official, addressing concerned farmers at the Midwest Organic and Sustainable Education Service conference earlier this year. That's where the law stands today.

Labeling Genetically Modified Organisms and Organic Products

The USDA strictly prohibits any genetically modified organisms from being labeled as "organic." Their production methods are defined as "a variety of methods to genetically modify organisms or influence their growth and development by means that are not possible under natural conditions or processes. Such prohibited methods include cell fusion, micro-encapsulation, macro-encapsulation, and recombinant DNA technology (including gene deletion, gene doubling, introducing a foreign gene, and changing the positions of genes when achieved by recombinant DNA technology)."

In the U.S., one of the ways organic farmers ensure that their products are free from GMOs is by avoiding genetically modified seeds or other materials when planting crops. They work with objective certifiers to implement preventative practices that effectively buffer their farms from GMO contamination.

So, with all of the hoo-haw revolving around consuming one hundred percent authentic organic products, why even bother? The answer is, of course, the quality and health saving benefits of eating superior products, while doing your part in protecting the environment. Study after study has shown:

1. **There is reduced exposure to pesticides and insecticides.** This is a significant benefit of organic produce.
2. **There is increased exposure to Omega-3 fatty acids.** Livestock fed through grazing usually has higher levels of Omega-3 fatty acids, which provide healthy heart benefits.

3. **There is less exposure to cadmium.** Studies have shown significantly lower levels of the toxic metal cadmium in organic grains.

4. **There are increased levels of vitamins, minerals, and antioxidants.** Organically grown fruits, vegetables, and grains have higher amounts of vitamin C, vitamin E, and carotenoids, as well as higher amounts of calcium, potassium, phosphorus, magnesium, and iron.

5. **Foods contain fewer bacteria.** Less exposure means less probability of bacteria in meat.

6. **There is less exposure to antibiotics.** Eating organic meat leads to less exposure to antibiotics and growth hormones that have been used to treat livestock. These medicines may lead to antibiotic resistance and other problems in humans.

7. **Nutrients.** Studies have shown moderate increases in some nutrients in organic produce, including flavonoids that have antioxidant properties.

8. **Omega-3 fatty acids.** Cattle feeding on primarily grass and alfalfa resulted in higher levels of Omega-3 fatty acids, a kind of fat that is more heart-healthy than other fats. Higher Omega-3 fatty acids are found in organic meats, dairy, and eggs.

9. **Toxic metal.** Cadmium is a toxic chemical naturally found in soil and absorbed by plants. When compared with conventionally grown crops, studies have shown significantly lower cadmium levels in organic grains, but not fruits and vegetables.

10. **Pesticide residue.** Compared with conventionally grown produce, organically grown produce has lower detectable levels of pesticide residue. Organic produce may have residue because of pesticides approved for

organic farming or because of airborne pesticides from conventional farms.

11. **Bacteria.** Meats produced conventionally may have a higher occurrence of bacteria resistant to antibiotic treatment. The overall risk of bacterial contamination of organic foods is the same as conventional foods.

What to Look for When You Buy Organic

If you're still awake and following the previous discussion about imported organic foods, you may be left with a queasy feeling. *Just how can lowly consumers make sound choices in buy-* 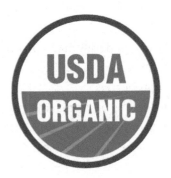 *ing organic foods in the United States?* Fear not. Overall, the regulation of organic foods is sound, as long as you look for the USDA Organic Seal. A 2002 law set in place a national organic foods standard. Foods labeled "USDA Organic" must adhere to the following standards:

- Produced in a way that protects natural resources
- Use only approved crops and livestock
- Refrain from crops and livestock that use genetic engineering (GMOs)
- Refrain from using ionizing radiation, sewage sludge, and most synthetic pesticides and fertilizers.

Fruits and vegetables where the organic label matters most are known as the "Dirty Dozen." Well, it's really the "Dirty Thirteen." They include:

The Dirty Dozen

Apples	Kale/Collard greens
Celery	Nectarines (imported)
Cherries	Peaches
Grapes	Pears
Hot peppers	Potatoes
Spinach	Strawberries
Tomatoes	

Fruits and vegetables that don't necessarily require you to buy organic are called the "Clean Fifteen."

The Clean Fifteen

Avocados	Kiwi
Asparagus	Mushrooms
Broccoli	Onions
Cabbage	Papayas
Cantaloupe	Pineapples
Cauliflower	Sweet corn*
Eggplants	Sweet peas (Frozen)
Honeydew melons	

The Cost of Buying Organic

There's no denying that buying organic products costs more than their traditionally grown counterparts. After all, producing delicious, healthy organic products costs farmers and suppliers more. Unfortunately, those costs are passed on to the consumer. Nevertheless, there are a few tips on how to save money when buying organic:

1. **Select foods from a variety of sources.** This gives you a better mix of nutrients and reduces your likelihood of exposure to a single pesticide.
2. **Buy fruits and vegetables in season whenever possible.** To get the freshest produce, ask your grocer what is in season or buy food from your local farmers market.
3. **Read food labels carefully.** Even though the label says a product is organic or contains organic ingredients, it doesn't necessarily mean it's a healthier alternative. Some organic products may still be high in sugar, salt, fat, or calories.
4. **Wash and scrub fresh fruits and vegetables thoroughly under running water.** Washing helps remove dirt, bacteria, and traces of chemicals from the surface of fruits and vegetables, but not all pesticide residues can be removed by washing. Discarding outer leaves of leafy vegetables can reduce contaminants. Peeling fruits and vegetables can remove contaminants, but may also reduce nutrients.

Where to Shop for Organic Food

Finding the best deals on organic food can often be an adventure. Unless you buy products from local growers, you'll need to research the best sources of organic food in your particular area. The good news is that once you find them, you can consider them a reputable food source and offer them your repeat business.

If you're new to an area or are new to the process of buying organic food, start with these handy online resources:

Location	Resource
United States	Eat Well Guide or Local Harvest
United Kingdom	FARMA
Australia	Australian Farmers' Markets Directory
Canada	Farmers' Markets in Canada

Summary - Why Should You Eat Organic?

Let's face it. Shopping for and buying organic food is much more trouble than grabbing a box of Fruit Loops off the shelf. It's supposed to be. Understanding how your food is grown and processed can have a major impact on your mental and emotional health as well as the environment. Organic foods are higher in beneficial nutrients (such as antioxidants) than conventionally processed foods, and they're better choices for people suffering from allergies to foods, chemicals, or preservatives.

Children and fetuses are particularly vulnerable to pesticide exposure because their immune systems have yet to mature.

Eating traditionally processed foods can lead to accumulated pesticide exposure. Their "body burden" over the years can lead to a variety of health issues such as headaches, birth defects, and added strain on the immune system. Studies have shown that consuming even low doses of pesticides can increase your risk for certain types of cancers including leukemia, lymphoma, brain tumors, breast, ovarian, and prostate cancer. Children and fetuses are particularly vulnerable to pesticide exposure because their immune systems have yet to mature, causing developmental delays, behavioral disorders, autism, immune system harm, and motor dysfunction.

Pregnant women are more vulnerable to the added stress that pesticides put on organs that are already working overtime to support their growing babies. Pesticides can be passed directly from the mother to the child in the womb, as well as through her breast milk.

Finally, organic farming is better for the environment. Organic farmers and growers reduce pollution, conserve water, reduce soil erosion, increase soil fertility, and use less energy while growing their crops.

In the next chapter, we'll discuss genetically modified organisms, genetically engineered foods, and how they can impact the production and sales of organic food. Stay tuned.

CHAPTER THREE

Genetically Modified Organisms

*Experience and extensive testing have shown that GE foods
have not lived up to their promise.*
–Steven Druker

Have you ever dreamed of eating a fluorescent pig?
How about salmon that glows in the dark or goat's
milk riddled with spider webs? You might be sur-
prised to learn *you already have.*

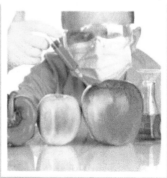

Humans have been domesti-
cating plants and animals for more
than 12,000 years, mostly through
selective and artificial breeding.
To this day, it's at the center of one
of the most controversial debates
in modern science, with as many
opponents as supporters. Why?

45

It's simple. People want to know what they're eating and if it's safe.

GMOs can lead to cancer and a host of other life-threatening diseases, and they're also bad for the environment. Unknown dangers lurk deep within ears of corn, tomatoes, and other popular foods, and should be labeled and federally mandated so consumers can decide for themselves whether or not they're going to pass on that box of Girl Scout cookies for a handful of raw carrots. But what actually constitutes genetic modifying isn't always clear.

At the most basic level, a genetically modified organism is any organism that has had its genes altered by either man or nature, in such a way that it does not occur naturally by mating or natural recombination. This *Frankenfood* is oftentimes easy to miss.

How It All Started

Genetically modifying organisms began by breeding animals across similar species. Examples include breeding a male donkey with a female horse to yield a mule, the beefalo (breeding a buffalo with a cow), and a bottlenose dolphin with a false killer whale that ends up as a wholphin. Then, things got interesting.

They argued that there has never been any evidence of health issues associated with GMOs and the impact on the environment is less harmful than traditional agriculture.

The most common way plants and animals are altered is by introducing the DNA from a bacteria, plant, virus, or animal "transgenically" into another organism. Genes can be taken from the cells of an existing organism, or one that's artificially synthesized. These days, genetically modifying organisms are so common, genes can be checked in and out of genetic libraries like library books.

One clever way scientists have fooled around with genetics is by removing the DNA of spiders and introducing them into that of a goat. The goat's milk is harvested, and the silk protein is isolated and extracted to make lightweight, ultra-strong material used in making artificial ligaments and tendons, bulletproof vests, and improved vehicular airbags.

Some genetically modified organisms are harmless and purely ornamental, such as flowers that are tweaked to produce various colors, shapes, and sizes. The bulk, however, are crops engineered by big food corporations that are supported by the opinions of the science community and the United States government.

The most famous genetic modifications started back in 1976 when the Monsanto Company created Roundup®, the brand name of a broad-spectrum, glyphosate-based herbicide to produce higher volumes of crops resistant to pests, insecticides, and fertilizers. More on that later.

Aside from larger agricultural companies (called BigAg), scientists are the most vocal in favor of creating and teasing GMOs. Biotech companies such as B.A.SF, Bayer, Monsanto, DuPont, Dow Chemical, and Syngenta (called The "Big Six"), have an unshakable faith in genetically engineered crops using their products. They hold major influence over mainstream media outlets and have close relationships with government agencies such as the U.S. Food and Drug Administration.

The goat's milk is harvested to make lightweight, ultra-strong material used in making artificial ligaments and tendons, bulletproof vests, and improved car airbags.

In June 2016, 129 Nobel Laureates in support of genetically modified organisms signed a letter urging anti-GMO organizations to abandon their campaign against GMOs. The group argued that there has never been any evidence of health issues associated with GMOs and the impact on the environment was less harmful than traditional agriculture. They also claimed that GMOs have the potential to reduce death and disease from issues in developing countries. The opponents weren't buying it.

On the flip-side are Greenpeace and Fairtrade International, leading the way in opposing GMOs. They claim that bioengineering is akin to playing Russian roulette with humans and their environment, fear that the risks GMOs pose are still unknown and may have unforeseeable environmental, social, and health impacts for years to come. "There is widespread public concern about the long-term effects of GMO crops," said Gelkha Buitrago, head of standards at Fairtrade International, with offices in Washington D.C., Manila, and Barcelona. "Contamination of conventional crops and wild plants, potential damage to wildlife, and the uncertain effects on human health when consuming these foods."

For the most part, commercial genetically modified crops are limited to cotton, soybeans, maize, and canola with traits that provide either herbicide tolerance or insect resistance. The problem is, they've crept into nearly every processed product on the market. Good luck trying to find a bag of Doritos that hasn't been tinkered with in one form or another.

How Genetically Modified Organisms Have Evolved Over Time

1973   Herbert Boyer and Stanley Cohen produced the first genetically modified organism: a bacteria-resistant to the antibiotic kanamycin

1974   Rudolf Jaenisch created a transgenic mouse by introducing foreign DNA into its embryo

1976   Original Roundup® brand herbicide commercialized for agricultural use in Canada

1978   The first genetically engineered, synthetic "human" insulin was produced using E.coli bacteria

1982   Eli Lilly sold the first commercially available biosynthetic human insulin under the brand name Humulin

1982   An antibiotic-resistant tobacco plant was produced making it the first genetically modified crop

1983   The first GMO plant was produced

1985   The first transgenic livestock was produced

1992   China became the first country to commercialize transgenic plants by introducing a virus-resistant tobacco

1994   The Flavr Savr tomato was released, making it the first commercialized genetically modified food

1996-2013   The total surface area of land cultivated with GM crops increased by a factor of one hundred

2000   Vitamin A-enriched golden rice was the first plant developed with increased nutrient value for third world countries

2003   GloFish, the first genetically modified animal was commercialized

2011	Green-fluorescent cats were created to help find therapies for HIV/AIDS and other diseases
2014	Soybeans accounted for half of all genetically modified crops planted in 2014
2015	AquAdvantage salmon became the first genetically modified animal to be approved for food use

Crops

The first generation of genetically modified crops was used for human food as well as feed for livestock and animals. It provided built-in resistance to pests, diseases, harsh environmental conditions, spoilage, and insecticides. The second generation focused on improving the quality of products by enhancing their nutrient profiles. The third generation of GMOs was used in non-food products such as pharmaceutical agents and biofuels. But it was the first generation of modified crops that caused all the hoo-haw.

The controversy started with Monsanto's Roundup® weed killer. In November 2012, the *Journal of Food and Chemical Toxicology* published a paper titled *Long Term Toxicity of Roundup Herbicide and a Roundup-Tolerant genetically modified maize*[26] by Gilles-Eric Séralini and his team of researchers at France's Caen University. It was the first of its kind under controlled conditions that examined the possible effects of a GMO maize diet treated with Monsanto's Roundup® herbicide.

In the study, one hundred female and one hundred male rats were used. Two of the groups were fed NK603, a variety of Roundup® Ready corn made by Monsanto that was deregulated in the U.S. in 2000 and commercialized in 2001

---

26 Republished study: Long-term toxicity of a Roundup herbicide and a Roundup-tolerant genetically modified maize - https://pubmed. ncbi.nlm.nih.gov/27752412/

under the brand name Roundup Ready 2®. The third group was given drinking water with the lowest permissible limit of Roundup®, and the fourth control group was fed a standard diet of the closest variety of non-GM maize.

More advanced research using fluorescent pigs has led to the study of human organ transplants, regeneration of ocular photoreceptor cells.

At the conclusion of the study, researchers found the rats that were fed NK603 or given water containing Roundup® died significantly earlier than the rats in the control group. They also developed hormonal and sex-related problems in females such as mammary tumors, pituitary, and kidney problems, while males died mostly from kidney failure. Up to fifty percent of the male rats and seventy percent of females died prematurely, compared with only thirty and twenty percent in the control group, respectively.

Séralini's study showed that ninety-day tests commonly used on GM foods by the FDA and BigAg are not nearly long enough to produce long-term side effects such as cancer, organ damage, and premature death. In Séralini's study, the first tumors didn't even appear until four to seven months into the study.

Agricultural development of GMOs has focused on three goals: Increased production, improved conditions for agricultural workers, and sustainability. Although GMOs have not always been embraced with open arms, science and government cling to the argument that genetically modified crops are beneficial to farmers through decreased use of pesticides and increased crop yields which result in higher profits. Many of these crops have been genetically modified to be resistant to selected herbicides—usually glyphosate or glufosinate-based products such as Monsanto's Roundup®. In the U.S., ninety-three percent of soybeans and most of the GM maize grown is glyphosate-tolerant.

Animals

Mammals have proven to be the best and closest models mimicking man and are vital to the development of new products, cures, and treatments for human diseases. As of 2018, there were only three approved genetically modified animals used for research: Goats, chickens, and salmon. Stable gene expressions have also been accomplished using rats, pigs, sheep, and other animals, so we'll have to wait and see what crazy ideas mad scientists come up with next.

Livestock has been one of the most aggressively studied animals by scientists. Important traits including milk composition, disease resistance, growth rate, meat quality, and survival have been significantly improved to the benefit of consumers and commercial applications.

More advanced research using fluorescent pigs has led to the study of human organ transplants and regeneration of ocular photoreceptor cells, although it's hard to imagine what the

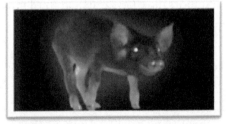

market would be for fluorescent pigs once they're done with the study. In 2011, green fluorescent cats were engineered in an effort to discover new therapies for HIV/AIDS and other immunodeficiency diseases. After the studies were completed, they went on to enjoy starring roles in science fiction thrillers that included *Curse of the Martian Virgins and Escape from Planet Voltar.*

Insects

Because of the significance of malaria in human health, scientists are constantly looking for ways to control the proliferation and types of mosquitos. One way is to engineer malaria-free mosquitos by inserting a gene that reduces the presence of the malaria parasite, then test the results by introducing them into high concentration areas such as Disneyland or backyard barbeques at your boss's house. Genetically modified mosquitos also help combat the life-threatening transmission of dengue fever.

The Contested Issue of GMOs

As with many other forms of new technology, support for GMOs can be polarizing: Those in favor of genetic engineering claim they offer enhanced medical, commercial, and scientific benefits not currently available. Opponents claim that even with the substantial advances made in GMO research, we still don't know enough about them to offer comfort and alternatives to the public.

Ever since the Marlboro Man ambled into town on horseback with a lung dart dangling from his lips, people simply don't trust what they're told.

Some of the most studied areas are in the agricultural and biological sciences, and has resulted in ample data to study. Scientists claim the data has yet to show anything risky or dangerous about using and consuming GMO products. The challenge is getting past the public's distrust of big business and the government. Ever since the Marlboro Man ambled into town on horseback with a lung dart dangling from his lips, people simply don't trust what they're told. They need ways to confirm it for themselves.

At the center of the controversy is Monsanto, the creators of Roundup Ready® crops. Monsanto also manufactured Agent Orange and DDT, two other "great ideas" they sold to the U.S. government during Operation Ranch Hand[27] in the Vietnam conflict. From 1961 to 1971, Agent Orange was responsible for more than 400,000 deaths and injuries of American soldiers and four million Vietnamese while deforesting Vietnam, Cambodia, and Laos, even though Monsanto promised there was no risk to human life while handling the lethal defoliant. Nevertheless, there are a few beneficial GMO exceptions, including the care and treatment of diabetics.

According to the Center for Disease Control and Prevention, more than thirty million people in the United States suffer from Type 1 and Type 2 diabetes, a staggering nine-plus percent of the population. Both types of diabetics can suffer from insufficient, naturally occurring insulin, a hormone that aids in blood glucose metabolism. Because they often suffer from a shortage of naturally-occurring insulin, millions of diabetics

---

27 Agent Orange. https://www.history.com/topics/vietnam-war/agent-orange-1

depend on manufactured insulin to manage their condition. Without it, how would they survive?

In 1889, two German researchers, Oskar Minkowski and Joseph von Mering, discovered that when the pancreas gland was removed from dogs, the animals suffered from symptoms of diabetes and died soon afterward. They hypothesized that the tiny pancreas was the site where insulin was produced. In 1982, Eli Lilly went on to sell the first commercially available biosynthetic human insulin under the brand name Humulin®.

There is mounting evidence that the insertion of even one gene into a cell's DNA alters the expression pattern of the genes throughout the entire cell.

Scientists argue that genetically modified products are tightly controlled. According to the Council for Biotechnology Information, whose members include B.A.SF, Bayer, Dow, DuPont Pioneer, Monsanto, and Syngenta, federal regulations require GMOs to pass more than seventy-five different safety tests. Each GMO takes an average of thirteen years and $130 million in research and development before it reaches the market. The rigorous testing and approval process means it's easier for the well-funded corporate sector to dominate the GMO market. The problem is, objective testing simply doesn't exist. As with organic food (see chapter three), most testing is funded by the companies with deep pockets who have the most to lose, so they deliberately influence the findings to support their line of business.

Claims Against GMOs

Similar to any other cause in today's political climate, GMOs foster as much controversy as they do good, largely because we're navigating upstream in uncharted waters without a paddle. Laypersons and scientists alike just don't know—or are willing to admit—how our actions today will impact human health tomorrow. According to the Fairfield, Iowa-based Institute for Responsible Technology (a group of anti-GMO activists), "Genetically modified foods have been linked to toxic and allergic reactions, sickness, sterile and dead livestock, and damage to virtually every organ studied in lab animals."

The Non-GMO Project[28] states, "Most developed nations do not consider GMOs to be safe. In more than sixty countries around the world, including Australia, Japan, and all of the countries in the European Union, there are significant restrictions or outright bans on the production and sale of GMOs."

The Top Twenty GMO Foods and Ingredients to Avoid

Aspartame   According to the U.S. Environmental Protection Agency, aspartame is a chemical that causes neurotoxicity[29]. Most notably, methanol is converted into formaldehyde. The U.S. Department of Labor considers formaldehyde a toxic and hazardous substance that should not be ingested. Recent research has demonstrated

---

28 The Non-GMO Project - https://www.nongmoproject.org/
29 https://globalhealing.com/natural-health/
health- dangers-of-aspartame/

the highly carcinogenic effects of aspartame consumption[30].

Corn   Several studies have shown regular dietary consumption of Bt-corn (maize), the GMO version of corn, leads to serious health concerns and negatively affects the kidney and liver (the dietary detoxifying organs), as well as in the heart, adrenal glands, and spleen.

Sugar beets   Sugar beets constitute nearly 130 million metric tons, or thirty-five percent of sugar, produced globally every year. Sugar beets are used to produce sucrose. In addition to glyphosate DNA, sugar beets are repeatedly coated with toxic chemicals during their growing cycle. It contains HFCS (High Fructose Corn Syrup) and is made from corn which is likely to be a GMO strain. Mercury has been found in HFCS as a result of the manufacturing process.

Soybeans   Soy has been associated with a wide range of health concerns, and GMO soy has been linked to pancreatic concerns. Soy lecithin is a waste product from the processing of crude soy oil, and typically contains solvents and pesticides.

Corn starch   The concerns with corn starch have been known about since the 1970s. Corn starch is a highly processed corn product made from genetically modified corn. It offers no nutritional value and carries all the dangers associated with GMO foods.

---

30 https://globalhealing.com/natural-health/
top-20-gmo-foods-and-ingredients-to-avoid/#references

Tomatoes   When tested, genetically modified tomatoes have been found to have less cancer-preventing antioxidant activity than their natural counterparts. The genetic modifications result in overall reduced nutritional value.

Sausage   Most sausage contains corn syrup or corn syrup solids, in addition to the other preservatives and likely contains a GMO.

Ice cream   Ice cream features a range of HFCS, corn syrup, and corn starch, plus rGBH[31].

Non-organic and synthetic vitamins
    Many vitamins, including top children's vitamins, use "vegetable" products as a base for the vitamin. Many of these "vegetables" come from corn and soy products, and many also contain aspartame and hydrogenate oils.

Infant formula
    Milk that contains rGBH and genetically modified soy constitute the foundation for most infant formulas unless they specifically state they are organic.

Beef   Beef feed may contain GMO alfalfa, corn, and soy.

Milk   Monsanto's recombinant Bovine Growth Hormone (rBGH) can be injected into cows to increase milk output.

Alfalfa   Although GMO alfalfa planting had been halted, as of 2013, GM alfalfa returned to the fields.

Vegetable oil   Vegetable oil typically comes from corn, soybean, cotton, or canola oils. All of these crops

---

31 ttps://www.organicvalley.coop/blog/
rBGH-decoded-what-is-bovine-growth-hormone/

have been genetically modified to withstand being doused by Roundup®.

Canola oil Contains rapeseed that has been genetically altered. As of 2009, ninety percent of Canada's rapeseed crop was herbicide-tolerant.

Margarine and shortening

 Another form of vegetable oil and contain all the GMO concerns that vegetable oils contain.

Hawaiian papaya

 This type of genetically modified papaya primarily affects those living on the West Coast. It contains DNA from the ringspot virus.

Squash Many squash varieties have been genetically modified to fight off the diseases that can affect them.

Flax GMO flax has been grown (illegally, for what it's worth) in Canada. Flax from Canada may be infected, as well as from many areas of the EU.

One of the most vocal opponents to GMOs is Steven Druker, a public interest attorney and the Executive Director of the Alliance for Bio-Integrity based in Salt Lake City. In 1998, rather than breaking into the FDA's offices in a modern-day Watergate, he initiated a lawsuit forcing the FDA to divulge the contents of its files on genetically engineered foods, followed by a book that detailed his experiences. "Experience and extensive testing have shown that GE foods have not lived up to their promise," says Druker. "In fact, they have abysmally failed. In many cases, they have reduced yields, not increased yields. They have dramatically increased herbicide use, they have not been benign to the environment, they've created environmental havoc, depletion of beneficial soil microbes. They have not produced food with enhanced nutritional profiles. They have not been producing food in a safe manner."

In his book[32], Druker describes how the commercialization of genetically engineered foods has led to fraudulent behavior on the part of the U.S. Food and Drug Administration and other government agencies, violating explicit federal food safety laws. Druker says, "FDA's falsehoods have been abundantly supplemented with falsehoods disseminated by eminent scientists and scientific institutions, and the entire GE food venture." The FDA's own scientists have long recognized the problems connected to genetically engineered foods and suppressed memos by their superiors who lied to the public.

Both sides have dug into trench warfare and are lobbing artillery shells back and forth at each other, while little changes in the technology or the ways it's communicated to the public.

The problem with current genetic engineering is based on the flawed assumption that a single gene will not impact the action of others, disrupting their normal functions. If you believe that, I have some wonderful Arizona beachfront land to sell you. In 2007, the *New York Times* published an article outlining how "the presumption that genes operate independently has been institutionalized since 1976 when the first biotech company was founded. In fact, it is the economic and regulatory foundation on which the entire biotechnology industry is built."

---

32 *Altered Genes, Twisted Truth: How the Venture to Genetically Engineer Our Food Has Subverted Science, Corrupted Government, and Systematically Deceived the Public*

The late David Schubert, Ph.D., a molecular biologist and the head of Cellular Neurobiology at the Salk Institute for Biological Studies in La Jolla, California, claimed in the journal *Nature Biotechnology*, "There is mounting evidence that the insertion of even one gene into a cell's DNA alters the expression pattern of the genes throughout the entire cell." He said, "Facts like these cast doubt on the soundness of agricultural bioengineering and entail the conclusion that it is not a safe option."

Summary

Unfortunately, both sides have dug into trench warfare and are lobbing artillery shells back and forth at each other, while little changes in the technology or the ways it's communicated to the public. On one hand, opponents of GMO-based food raise a good point: We simply don't know what years of consuming GMOs is going to do to our health. Even though it's been over fifty years since its inception, there are still no long-term human studies to support either side of the controversy. And it's not likely to change any time soon, despite heavy pressure from organizations such as the Non-GMO Project.

There's simply too much money at stake. The Big Six agrochemical companies have spent millions to ensure nothing changes in the way they currently do business. As you'll read in the next chapter, the government and big business have discovered even more opaque ways to confuse consumers by coming up with indecipherable labels even they don't understand.

It's going to be a long, hard battle.

CHAPTER FOUR

GMOs, Legislation, and the Business of Cancer

I tried many different cigarettes. I chose Camels for their flavor and for their cool, cool mildness - pack after pack!
–John Wayne cigarette ad

At the close of World War II, thousands of randy young soldiers hooked on cigarettes anxiously returned home, ready to begin their new lives. The government, big business, and Madison Avenue were ready for them.

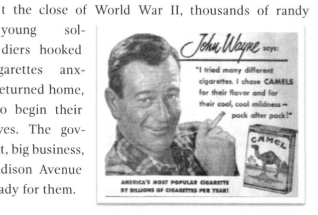

Big tobacco was one of the first shams designed to guarantee that consumers remained addicted to their products without knowing how lethal they really were. Granted, you don't have to be a rocket scientist to figure out that inhaling a butt of burning weeds isn't good for you, but people didn't seem to care. They still don't.

The tobacco industry demonstrated an utter disregard for the health of the very people who made them rich while being bilked out of their hard-earned money through a series of strategically designed cover-ups, accompanied by out-and-out dishonesty. These tobacco companies included Philip Morris International, Altria, British American Tobacco, Imperial Brands, Japan Tobacco International, and ITC Limited, and are the same companies that serve as role models for the current controversy over GMOs that are currently gripping our society.

At the front of the GMO squabbles are Bayer, B.A.SF, Dow AgroScience, Dupont Pioneer, Monsanto, and Syngenta, also known as the "Big Six" biotech companies. They're in the business of selling seed and herbicides to farmers embroiled in the debate over GMOs. This is largely because of their government lobbying skills, and their ability to influence GMO regulations and practices that farmers depend on for government subsidies. The Big Six claim they're engaging in open conversations on the subject of GMOs. The public disagrees and is right to question their motives and acts. These companies are putting profitability above everything else, including public health and the environment.

What's become obvious is their blatant disregard for protecting the public's health while producing their products. Large bio-agriculture companies are more concerned with their bottom line—budgets, sales, overhead costs, and profit—than they are about serving the consumer with a safe and healthy product.

There are several key aspects currently affecting the way large agricultural companies are able to conduct business and in turn affect us the consumers: GMOs (with and without pesticides), legislation, and the business of cancer.

Genetically Modifying Organisms

As with any successful businesses, government and agriculture companies are motivated by the bottom line: How much money can they earn from farmers and consumers while pushing inferior products? One early example was Aspartame®.

Since 1974, Aspartame® has been sold as an artificial sweetener 200 times sweeter than table sugar, and sold under brand names including NutraSweet® and Equal®. After enjoying massive popularity with consumers, scientists discovered that Aspartame® caused neurotoxicity and produced formaldehyde—a toxic ingredient banned by the U.S. Department of Labor. It was also associated with serious health problems, including cancer, cardiovascular disease, Alzheimer's disease, seizures, stroke, and dementia, as well as negative effects that included intestinal dysbiosis, mood disorders, headaches, and migraines.

Large bio-agriculture companies are more concerned with their bottom line—budgets, sales, overhead costs, and profit—than they are about serving the consumer with a safe and healthy product.

Both FDA and independent scientists raised concerns about the health effects and shortcomings in the science submitted to the FDA by the manufacturer, G.D. Searle. (Monsanto bought Searle in 1984)[33]. In 1987, UPI[34] published a series of articles reporting these concerns, including Aspartame's® link to health problems, the poor quality of industry funded research that ultimately led to its approval, and the revolving door relationships between FDA officials and the food industry.

Researchers in the U.S. who attempt to test the safety of GMOs are routinely ostracized by the rank-and-file industry. It's even worse for public action groups that include the Organic Consumers Association, the Non-GMO Project, Are We Eating Fishy Food, GMO Inside, and Just Label It!. Ironically, it's not the same in Europe. Europe simply doesn't allow GMOs in their food to the extent that the U.S. does. Nevertheless, they still label it.

To make matters worse, any corporation that wants to conduct its own scientific study to determine whether or not its product is safe receives blessings from the FDA and the EPA to hire its own scientific research team, use that team to conduct, record and submit that analysis to the EPA. Common sense tells anyone that it's a bald-faced violation in the face of an independent study of the products.

Let's face it. America is a super-size nation. It's all about quantity, not quality. How much money can we make by selling questionable products and. . .*would you like fries with that?* It's more important for CEOs at the top of the food chain to

---

33 Aspartame: Decades of Science Point to Serious Health Risks https://usrtk.org/sweeteners/aspartame_health_risks/

34 UPI investigative report: NutraSweet: Questions swirl https://www.upi.com/Archives/1987/10/12/UPI-investigative-report-NutraSweet-Questions-swirl/5886561009600/

be able to buzz around in their Lear jets than it is to admit to the public the sources of their exorbitant salaries. What most of the public doesn't know (and perhaps, couldn't really care less about) is that in addition to their exorbitant salaries, these CEOs receive and give away in the form of contributions and gifts a series of share options and other hidden goldmines so the elite rich—the top five percent—can continue to squirrel away their loot. We'll talk about GMOs more in chapter four.

The Legislation

After years of finagling, American food manufacturers are now required to alert consumers to the presence of genetically modified ingredients through labels, QR codes, or text messages. In reality though, who wants to take the time to extensively research the bag of carrots in their hand while they're shopping for produce, and do they even own a smartphone with internet access so they can scan the QR code or follow the link on the label? And, just to make things more confusing for consumers, manufacturers have changed the name from "genetically engineered" or "genetically modified organism" to "bioengineered food" to describe organisms that scientists created by tweaking their DNA. It's a mess.

We already know that Monsanto has caused deaths. Their history with Agent Orange and their current involvement with GMOs has made that clear.

Most consumers have no idea what "bioengineered food" means and associate it with some form of "Six Million

Dollar Man" created in a laboratory. The term applies to foods containing detectable genetic material that has been modified through lab techniques and cannot be created through conventional breeding or found in nature. (Their words, not mine). This includes genetic traits that include resistance to certain pesticides. The disclosure requirement took effect on January 1, 2020, though compliance won't be mandatory until January 1, 2022.

In the ruling, the USDA lists the ingredients that manufacturers must disclose unless records demonstrate that they are not bioengineered. The list initially consisted of genetically modified alfalfa, apples, canola, corn, cotton, eggplant, and papaya that is resistant to the ringspot virus, pink flesh pineapple, potatoes, salmon, soybeans, sugar beets, and summer squash. The USDA plans to revise the list annually.

In November 2012, some of America's most profitable chemical companies teamed up with a handful of large food corporations, and spent more than $45 million in advertising to stop Proposition 37, a California initiative to require labeling of genetically modified foods. At the time, it was only the third state to put a measure on a ballot for GMO labeling.

We already know that Monsanto has caused deaths. The company's history with Agent Orange and its current involvement with GMOs has made that clear. Monsanto was the No. 1 against the proposition with a single contribution of $8,112,867 to ensure that the proposition did not pass. The second highest contributor was Dupont at $5,400,000, followed by Pepsi with $2,145,400. You don't have to be Warren Buffett to figure out who represents the most shameless conflicts of interest between consumers and cancer research and treatment.

According to Ballotpedia[35], had California's Proposition 37 passed, the legislation would have:

- Required labeling on raw or processed food offered for sale to consumers if made from plants or animals with genetic material changed in specified ways.
- Prohibited labeling or advertising such food, or other processed food, as "natural."
- Exempted foods that were: certified organic; unintentionally produced with genetically engineered material; made from animals fed or injected with genetically engineered material but not genetically engineered themselves; processed with or containing only small amounts of genetically engineered ingredients; administered for treatment of medical conditions; sold for immediate consumption, as in a restaurant; or alcoholic beverages.

The competition was fierce, with each side putting their money where their disagreements were. Arguments in favor of the proposition listed in the state's official voter guide[36] included:

- "You should have the right to know what's in your food."
- "You'll have the information you need about foods that some physicians and scientists say are linked to allergies and other significant health risks."
- "Over forty countries around the world require labels for genetically modified foods."

---

35 Ballotpedia - https://ballotpedia.org/California_Proposition_37,_Mandatory_Labeling_of_Genetically_Engineered_Food_ (2012)

36 California Voter Guide (official) - https://ballotpedia.org/California_Voter_Guide_(official)

Donors in Favor of Proposition 37

Donor	Amount
Organic Consumers Fund	$1,334,865
Mercola Health Resources	$1,115,000
Kent Whealy	$1,000,000
Nature's Path Foods	$660,709
Dr. Bronner's Magic Soaps	$566,438
Mark Squire/Stillonger Trust	$440,000
Wehah Farm (Lundberg Family Farms)	$251,500
Ali Partovi	$219,113
Amy's Kitchen	$200,000
Great Foods of America	$177,000
Alex Bogusky	$100,000
Clif Bar & Co.	$100,000
Cropp Cooperative (Organic Valley)	$100,000
Annie's, Inc.	$50,000
Michael S. Funk	$50,000
Nutiva	$50,000

Opposition to Proposition 37 was fervent. Compared to the limited resources in support of Proposition 37, huge biotech and food companies with deep pockets overwhelmed their opposition's efforts.

Donors in Opposition of Proposition 37

Donor	Amount
Monsanto	$8,112,867
E.I. Dupont De Nemours & Co.	$5,400,000
Pepsico, Inc.	$2,145,400
Grocery Manufacturers Association	$2,002,000
DOW Agrisciences	$2,000,000
Bayer Cropscience	$2,000,000
B.A.SF Plant Science	$2,000,000
Syngenta Corporation	$2,000,000

Kraft Foods Global	$1,950,500
Coca-Cola North America	$1,700,500
Nestle USA	$1,315,600
Conagra Foods	$1,176,700
General Mills	$1,135,300
Kellogg Company	$790,000
Smithfield Foods	$683,900
Del Monte Foods	$674,100
Campbell's Soup	$500,000
Heinz Foods	$500,000
Hershey Company	$493,900
The J.M. Smucker Company	$485,000
Bimbo Bakeries	$422,900
Ocean Spray Cranberries	$387,100
Mars Food North America	$376,650
Council for Biotechnology Information	$375,000
Hormel Foods	$374,300
Unilever	$372,100
Bumble Bee Foods	$368,500
Sara Lee	$343,600
Kraft Food Group	$304,500
Pinnacle Foods	$266,100
Dean Foods Company	$253,950
Biotechnology Industry Organization	$252,000
Bunge North America	$248,600
McCormick & Company	$248,200
Wm. Wrigley Jr. Company	$237,664
Abbott Nutrition	$234,500
Cargill, Inc.	$226,846
Rich Products Corporation	$225,537
Flowers Foods	$182,000
Dole Packaged Foods	$171,261
Knouse Foods Cooperative	$164,731

The opposition argued:

- "It's a deceptive, deeply flawed food labeling scheme that would add more government bureaucracy and taxpayer costs, create new frivolous lawsuits, and increase food costs by billions without providing any health or safety benefits."
- "It's full of special interest exemptions."
- "It authorizes shakedown lawsuits."

The Election Results

California Proposition 37

Result	Votes	Percentage
No	**6,442,371**	**51.4%**
Yes	6,088,714	48.6%

Win, lose or draw, transparency is our inalienable right. Yet, a handful of bloated companies including Monsanto, Kraft, Kellogg's, and General Mills have managed to escape while hiding critical information from consumers about the quality of our food for over twenty years.

The Grocery Manufacturers Association, which is composed of twelve companies including Pepsi, General Mills, and Conagra, have members on the boards of hospitals that are leaders in cancer research and treatment. It was founded in 1908 as the Grocery Manufacturers of America and headquartered in Washington, D.C. In September 2019, it announced that it would relaunch itself as the Consumer Brands Association effective January 2020.

Grocery Manufacturers Association Members

Archer Daniels Midland Company	Mars, Incorporated
Campbell Soup Company	Monsanto
Coca-Cola Company	B.A.SF
Dole Packaged Foods Company	Bayer
General Mills, Inc.	Dow
Kellogg Company	Syngenta

In 2013, the same companies raised millions of dollars to defeat a similar initiative in Washington state, followed by Oregon and Colorado in 2014.

List of Top 20 Right to Know Opponents

	Donor	No On 37[37]	No on 522[38]	No on 92[39]	No on 105[40]
1	Monsanto Co.	$8,112,867	$5,374,411	$5,958,750	$4,755,878
2	Dupont	$5,400,000	$3,880,159	$4,928,150	$3,000,000
3	PepsiCo	$2,485,400	$2,352,966	$2,350,000	$1,650,000
4	Grocery Manufacturers Association	$2,002,000	$11,000,000**	$169,190	$106,600
5	Kraft Foods	$2,000,500	-	$870,000	$1,030,000
6	B.A.SF Plant Science	$2,000,000	$500,000	-	-
7	Bayer CropScience	$2,000,000	$591,654	-	-
8	DOW $ Agrosciences	2,000,000	$591,654	$1,157,150	$306,500
9	Syngenta Corporation	$2,000,000	-	-	-
10	Coca-Cola N.A.	$1,690,500	$1,520,351	$1,170,000	$1,108,000
11	Nestle USA	$1,461,600	$1,528,206	-	-
12	General Mills	$1,230,300	$869,271	$695,000	$820,000
13	ConAgra Foods	$1,176,700	$828,251	$350,000	$250,000
14	Kellogg's Company	$790,700	$322,050	$500,000	250,000
15	Smithfield Foods	$683,900	-	-	$250,000

37 California
38 Washington
39 California
40 Oregon

16	Delmonte Foods	$674,100	$125,677	-	-
17	Campbell Soup Company	$598,000	$384,888	-	-
18	Smucker Company	$555,000	$349,978	$295,000	$345,000
19	Hershey Company	$518,900	$360,450	$320,000	$380,000
20	Biotechnology Industry Organization	$502,000	-		

Fortunately, states haven't thrown in the towel yet when it comes to voting for GMO right to know legislation. Here's a snapshot of what's currently pending in the legislature[41]:

Current Right to Know Activity by State

State	Action
Arizona	GMO-Free Phoenix
California	California Right to Know
Colorado	GMO-Free Colorado
Connecticut	Northeast Organic Farming Association, CT Chapter (Proposed Bill: HB 5117)
Florida	Label GMO Florida
Hawaii	Label It Hawaii (Proposed Bill: HB 2034/ SB 2443)
Idaho	GMO-Free Idaho
Illinois	GMO Free Illinois
Massachusetts	Northeast Organic Farming Association, MA Chapter (Proposed Bill: H3276)
Michigan	No GMO 4 Michigan
Minnesota	Right to Know Minnesota (Proposed Bill: S.F. 2563)
New Jersey	Label GMOs in New Jersey (Proposed Bill: HB 1367)

41 Just Label It! http://www.justlabelit.org/press-center/press-items/gmo-labeling-isnt-dead-see-which-states-are-leading-the-fight/

New York	www.gmofreeny.org
	info@gmofreeny.org
	www.facebook.com/gmofreeny
	www.twitter.com/gmofreeny
North Carolina	(Proposed Bill: HB 446)
Ohio	GMO Free Ohio
Oregon	GMO Free Oregon (Proposed Bills: SB 517 & HB 3346)
Utah	GMO Free Utah
Vermont	Vermont Right to Know GMO (Proposed Bill: HB 722)
Virginia	(Proposed Bill: HB 606)
Washington	Label It Washington (Bill Title: HB 2637)

The Business of Cancer

There is a strong relationship between business and cancer. Corporations spend millions of dollars surreptitiously keeping consumers in the dark while appointing big business executives to the board of directors at organizations such as the City of Hope. One well-known example is Michael Taylor, the former Food and Drug Administration Deputy Commissioner for Foods and Veterinary Medicine who also happens to be Monsanto's former Vice President for Public Policy. While at the FDA, he was instrumental in getting approval for Monsanto's genetically engineered bovine growth hormone.

Owners and top-level management routinely lie to the public that they're not motivated by money, yet are hauling in millions of dollars through company share options. Sitting on the boards of hospitals and cancer centers helps to control and ensure shareholder equity and not so much to help or cure cancer. We live in a world where corporations even control our treatment and cancer prevention. Having the same entities that are causing cancer tasked with treating it is a conflict of interest. Don't believe it? Then why did twenty out of thirty-two companies whose executives sit on the Board of Directors of the City of Hope vote against labeling for GMOs?

To ensure their anonymity, companies create smaller off-shoots hidden within the organization, using different names so they can claim they're not associated with the parent company. For instance, members of Pacific Northwest Food Industries are associated with the City of Hope. Other parent companies associated with "invisible" sub-companies include:

Haggens's Foods
Safeway, Inc.
Associated Grocers
Unified Grocers
Bimbo Bakeries
Pepsi-Cola Bottling Co.
Kraft Food
Kellogg's
Wrigley Sales
McCormick
ConAgra
General Mills
Ocean Spray
Sara Lee
Unified Western Grocers

Government Farm Subsidies

Government farm subsidies are government-supported financial benefits paid to a specific industry—in this case, agribusiness. These subsidies help reduce the risk farmers endure from dynamics such as the weather, commodities brokers, and disruptions in demand. If farmers' crops fail, their subsidies kick in to ensure that they'll make their bottom line. It sounds great. Who wouldn't want a way to make money without doing anything? It *is* great, but only until you read the fine print.

The federal government spends more than $20 billion a year on subsidies for farming businesses. Yet, only thirty-nine percent of the nation's more than two million farms receive these subsidies, with the lion's share of the handouts going to the largest producers of corn, soybeans, wheat, cotton, and rice.

They're discouraged from innovating, cutting costs, diversifying their land use, and taking other actions needed to prosper in the competitive economy.

Farmers' dependence on subsidies is the principal reason why the FDA yields so much power associated with large corporations making sure that the public doesn't understand what all GMOs encompass. Since the government holds the purse strings, it's in a position to dictate to farmers what they can and cannot do, and forces them to abide by a strict set of guidelines that usually don't support efforts for GMO transparency.

The History of Farm Subsidies[42]

1862 The Homestead Act in 1862 granted land in the West to settlers willing to farm it. The Morrill Act of 1862 funded colleges of agriculture. The Federal Farm Loan Act made government loans available to farmers. It also made sure there was enough food during World War I.

---

42 Agricultural Subsidies - https://www.downsizinggovernment. org/agriculture/subsidies

1887 The Hatch Act of 1887 funded agricultural research and the Smith-Lever Act of 1914 for agricultural education.

1916 The Federal Farm Loan Act of 1916 created cooperative banks to provide loans to farmers.

1929 The Agricultural Marketing Act of 1929 created the Federal Farm Board. It tried to keep crop prices from crashing. It became the Farm Credit Administration in 1933.

1933 Congress signed the Agricultural Adjustment Act. It paid farmers to reduce crop output. It doubled crop prices by 1937, and was overturned by the Supreme Court in 1936 because it taxed processors but gave funds to farmers.

1934 The Soil Conservation and Domestic Allotment Act paid farmers to plant soil-building crops, including beans and grasses, to counteract the drought.

1935 The Resettlement Administration trained farmers and adjusted farm debt payments. It also relocated farmers onto better land and taught them modern conservation and farming techniques.

1937 The Farm Tenancy Act created the Farmers' Home Corporation to provide loans for tenant farmers to buy their farms.

1938 The New Agricultural Adjustment Act remedied the 1933 AAA. This price support system lasted until the 1990s. The federal government guaranteed farmers a high enough price to remain profitable, and paid them to make sure the supply did not exceed demand.

1940- 1980 Congress considered farm policy reforms occasionally, usually when commodity prices were high, but then reverted to subsidy expansions when prices were lower

1996 Congress enacted reforms under the Freedom to Farm law, which allowed farmers greater flexibility in planting and increased reliance on market supply and demand.

2002 Congress enacted a farm bill that further reversed the 1996 reforms. The law increased projected subsidy payments, added new crops to the subsidy rolls, and created a new price guarantee scheme called the countercyclical program.

2014 Congress ended the direct payment program and the countercyclical program. It expanded the largest farm subsidy program—crop insurance—and added two new subsidy programs, the Agriculture Risk Coverage (ARC) program and the Price Loss Coverage (PLC) program.

Federal aid for crop farmers is deep and comprehensive. In addition to subsidizing and protecting farmers against the dynamic fluctuations in prices, revenues, tariff wars, and crop yields, it supports their conservation efforts, insurance coverage, marketing, export sales, research, and other activities.

Unfortunately, to continue qualifying for subsidies, farmers have to walk the straight and narrow, which is dictated by the FDA. They're discouraged from innovating, cutting costs, diversifying their land use, and taking other actions needed to prosper in the competitive economy.

Out of all the crops that farmers grow, the government only subsidizes corn, soybeans, wheat, cotton, and rice. Most of the direct aid goes to producers of these crops, not to livestock producers or fruit and vegetable growers. Guess who those are?

———————————————

Farming is a rough business. The number of people in the farming industry has slowly declining for decades. Nevertheless, it contributes more than $132.8 billion to the American economy and is in a huge state of transition. Smart technology is changing the way farmers work in agriculture and how Americans interact with their food. But will the FDA and other government subsidies play nice with these inevitable changes, which include GMO food labeling? According to a recent article in *Business Insider: Nine mind-blowing facts about the U.S. farming industry*[43]:

1. Agriculture's $1.053 trillion contributions to the U.S. economy is higher than the GDP of Indonesia.
2. While there are more than 2.6 million farms across the U.S., farmers and ranchers make up just over one percent of the labor force, compared to 1840 when workers in the agriculture industry made up seventy percent of the American workforce.
3. The local food market in the U.S. is expected to hit $20.2 billion, nearly doubling from 2014 to 2019, yet in 2017, the global market research company Mintel found "widespread mistrust" among consumers in how food is made.
4. Soybeans account for sixty percent of America's $23 billion worth of agricultural exports to China. The Chinese domesticated the soybean 3,000 years ago. It's heavily used for cooking oils and as feed for livestock. China has recently halted imports of American soybeans amid the escalating trade war with the U.S.
5. Extreme weather is the cause of ninety percent of crop losses in the U.S. Record-breaking cold temperatures in January, followed by intense snowfall in February and

---

43 9 mind-blowing facts about the US farming industry - https://markets.businessinsider.com/news/stocks/farming-industry-facts-us-2019-5-1028242678#

massive snowmelt in the spring led to flooding in the Midwest that may have cost the U.S. as much as $3 billion as pastures and crops were submerged underwater. In the West, total losses from the wildfires in Northern and Southern California have topped $12 billion. In the South, Texas A&M AgriLife Extension Service economists reported last year's Hurricane Harvey caused more than $200 million in crop and livestock losses.

6. Over 50,000 jobs in agriculture are available per year in the U.S., yet there aren't enough qualified graduates to fill the spots. In addition to working in the field, new hires may find themselves in a lab, an office, or perhaps even an open-concept, co-working space.

7. Soon, you'll be able to scan the sticker on an apple and trace its history as it made its way to your grocery basket. Smart labels are meant to assuage fears consumers may have about where their food comes from. They also target consumers who predominantly shop at local farmers' markets and want to make sure the food they buy at the store doesn't carry a significant carbon footprint.

8. Forty-one percent of the contiguous U.S. is used to feed livestock. That's 800 million acres; roughly the size of India. A study by *Bloomberg*[44] found that while U.S. agricultural land takes up 391 million acres—a fifth of the land in the forty-eight contiguous states—only 77.3 million of those acres are used to grow the food we eat.

9. Once a place to talk shop, #AgTwitter has helped curb depression among farmers. According to *PBS NewsHour*[45],

44 Here's How America Uses Its Land - https://www.bloomberg.com/graphics/2018-us-land-use/

45 For farmers, talking about mental health used to be taboo. Now there's #AgTwitter - https://www.pbs.org/newshour/nation/for-farmers-talking-about-mental-health-used-to-be-taboo-now-theres-agtwitter

rural areas have had some of the highest suicide rates of any geographic area in the United States. Suicide rates among farmers and agricultural workers outnumbered homicide rates between 1992 and 2010.

Summary

The important thing to remember is that not all GMOs are bad. The harmful ones are the ones that load corn, soy, and numerous other vegetables with pesticides, herbicides, and insecticides, attempting to go undetected. Even if you don't like the idea of genetically modifying plants, the public needs to know the truth. Government and agriculture are motivated by how much money they can make off of farmers and consumers by pushing low-quality products while hiding information under the surface, information that's exposed by product labeling.

GMOs that are simply clones of the original food can play a significant role in the ever-increasing war against world hunger and diabetes. Unfortunately, laws banning destructive products that contain toxic herbicides are not going to take place any time soon. So until things change, your best bet is to avoid them. Vote with your wallet to express your opinions about current food production and labeling practices.

---

*Farming is a rough business. The number of people
in the farming industry has been slowly declining for decades.*

Shop at markets such as Sprouts and Whole Foods markets. If you choose to stick with large-scale, "Top Ten" alternatives are Ralphs, Stater Brothers, Albertsons, Safeway, Vons, Food for Less, Publix, Smart and Final, Aldi Walmart, and Target. Try to shop exclusively in the organic food section. If you don't, you'll find yourself wandering through the center aisles that contain highly processed foods. There are no organic alternatives for Cocoa Puffs, hot dogs, or Pop-Tarts. Let me repeat that: There are no organic alternatives for Cocoa Puffs, hot dogs, or Pop-Tarts. You're eating GMOs.

Looking forward, as long as food companies and big biotech control the government and the farms, there won't be any honest scientific research. But at least we can hope.

In the next chapter, we'll look at how government and big businesses are attempting to regulate GMO food labeling and how it impacts your life.

CHAPTER FIVE

Regulation and the Cause for GMO Food Labeling

R egardless of which side you butter your bread, product labeling is one of the most hotly contested issues concerning regulators of genetically modified
products—whether or not they should be labeled and what
information labels should contain. Opponents of genetically
modified foods claim that scientists are "playing God" with
the products we consume. Others are already clamoring to
"patenting life" issues by claiming
intellectual property rights of new
offspring.

Even the broad, generic term has
come under fire. Regulators have
muddied the waters by taking it upon
themselves to change the commonly

accepted term "genetically modified organism" to "bioengineered food" just when the public has begun to warm up to the campaign.

Opponents claim GMO labeling guidelines really aren't necessary since they already exist. *Good luck trying to find them.* Others want you to believe that if GMOs were really dangerous, the FDA wouldn't label them at all—they'd simply pull them from the shelves. Still, others fear that labels spread fear and misinformation to consumers that could potentially drive up the price of food.

To make matters worse, consumers and federal regulators can't agree on exactly what should be included in labels. They run the gamut from the country of origin, ingredients that pose risks to some people (such as peanuts and gluten), as well as ingredients such as salt that most health authorities agree we should all limit. However, most do concur that consumers have a right to know whether or not the products they buy are grown using herbicide-intensive agriculture. At the same time, the American Medical Association and the American Association for the Advancement of Science take the position that absent scientific evidence of harm, even voluntary labeling is misleading and will falsely alarm consumers.

So, we're back to square one.

If GMOs are really safe, why do food companies keep hiding them from us?

Where Labeling Stands Today

Labeling of GMO products in the U.S. and Canada is voluntary, while countries in the European Union mandate that all food, including processed food or animal feed containing just under one percent and higher of approved GMOs must be labeled. The result has led to international trade disputes, litigation, and protests.

In the past, scientists and companies responded to the challenge by lobbying against GMO labeling in hopes that burying the technology would ultimately limit public concern[46]. They were wrong. Failure to label products made with GMOs only stoked the fires it was intended to quash. Questions started to immerge in the face of strong scientific consensus that GMOs are safe, a position supported by so-called unbiased sources including the World Health Organization[47] and the U.S. National Academies of Sciences, Engineering, and Medicine[48]. But by hiding the science from the public, people began questioning it even more. Their concerns were exacerbated by fears about GMO safety, clouded by questionable business practices.

Experience has shown that clear, simple GMO labeling helps to assuage questions and confusion by consumers. In July 2016, the state of Vermont required foods made with GMOs or their byproducts be labeled, "Produced with genetic engineering" or "Partially produced with genetic engineering." Contrary to people's expectations, consumers didn't stop buying GMO products. In fact, a 2018 study showed Vermonters

---

46 American Association for the Advancement of Science: 20 October 2012 - https://www.aaas.org/sites/default/files/AAAS_GM_statement.pdf

47 World Health Organization: Frequently asked questions on genetically modified foods - https://www.who.int/foodsafety/areas_work/food-technology/faq-genetically-modified-food/en/

48 U.S. National Academies of Sciences, Engineering, and Medicine - Genetically Engineered Crops

grew less opposed to GMOs, and sentiment for the products actually improved.

The fly in the ointment is there's no penalty
for failure to comply with the law.

The problem is, there are plenty of opportunities for scurrilous companies opposed to transparent labeling practices to bury information, confirming their products contain GMOs or ingredients made from them. Instead of requiring a simple symbol or text disclosure, the USDA rule allows companies to get away with workarounds such as QR codes, hyperlinks, and toll-free phone numbers to cloud their use of genetic engineering—all of which makes it impossible for consumers standing the in the produce department, holding a bag of carrots to answer, "Which of these bags should I buy?"

Equally worrisome is the rule's definition of bioengineered (BE) products—its proxy term for GMOs. The term is so lax that it allows thousands of products to avoid mandatory labeling even though they are all genetically engineered by any definition of the term.

A review of the literature[49][50] supports the scientific consensus that food made from GM crops poses no more risk to humans than conventionally produced food, but each product must be evaluated on a case by case basis. Big tobacco compa-

---

49 Statement by the AAAS Board of Directors On Labeling of Genetically Modified Foods: http://www.aaas.org/sites/default/files/AAAS_GM_statement.pdf

50 AMA Report on Genetically Modified Crops and Foods
January 2001 https://www.isaaa.org/kc/Publications/htm/articles/Position/ama.htm

nies said the same thing about cigarettes, and look what happened to them.

In 2016, congress passed the National Bioengineered Food Disclosure Standard (NBFDS). The law requires the USDA to establish a labeling standard for all genetically modified or bioengineered food. The decision was followed by a hard-fought battle by consumer groups that argued USDA regulations were purposely written in a manner that made them impossible to understand. Critics argued that companies weren't required to say they contained GMOs, noting instead that it's "bioengineered food." Even worse, food production companies still aren't required to label highly refined ingredients that come from GMO crops such as cane sugar, corn syrup, and processed vegetable oil.

Large food production companies are also not required to label highly refined ingredients that come from GMO crops, as long as there's no evidence of genetically engineered material. That means ingredients such as cane sugar, corn syrup, and processed vegetable oil can escape the labeling process, or labeled on a strictly voluntary basis. The National Milk Producers Federation stated that it was "pleased" with the USDA's decision to not require labels for milk produced by animals that consume bioengineered feed.

The requirements of the NBFDS were originally set to take effect by July 2018, but the USDA extended it for two years after a public comment period. They implemented it to take effect at the beginning of 2020, and required food companies to comply no later than January 1, 2022. The fly in the ointment is that there's no penalty for failure to comply with the law, which is in contrast to the USDA's National Organic Program that levies fines of up to $11,000 per violation.

Fortunately, the regulation makes allowances for organic products, so organic companies are not unnecessarily burdened to comply with the regulation. To make it easier on organic production, the final GMO labeling rule allows certified organic products to use absence claims that include "*not* genetically engineered" and "*non*-GMO." But there's a catch.

CRISPR-Cas9 Technology Emerges

The new law also exempts GMO ingredients developed through techniques such as CRISPR-Cas9 technology. Haven't heard of it? Believe me, you will.

CRISPR, (pronounced "crisper") stands for "clusters of regularly interspaced short palindromic repeats" and is shorthand for "CRISPR-Cas9," a simple yet powerful tool for editing genomes. It allows scientists to alter DNA sequences modifying their gene functions to correct genetic defects that include cystic fibrosis, cataracts, and Fanconi anemia, and also preventing the spread of diseases and improving the quality of crops. The CRISPR-Cas9 technique was first demonstrated by Rodolphe Barrangou and a team of researchers at Danisco, a food ingredients company based in Copenhagen.

The CRISPR-associated protein Cas9 is an enzyme that acts similarly to a pair of "molecular scissors," capable of cutting strands of DNA. CRISPR-Cas9 technology was originally adapted from the natural defense mechanisms of bacteria. Cas9 enzymes use CRISPR-derived RNA to foil attacks from viruses and other foreign bodies by excising and destroying DNA from foreign invaders. When Cas9 enzymes are transferred into other organisms, they allow for manipulation, or "editing" genes. CRISPR-Cas9 technology is also being used to engineer probiotic cultures (in yogurt, for example) and to vaccinate industrial cultures against viruses. As with its predecessors, it is also being used in crops to improve yield, drought tolerance, and nutritional properties.

These exemptions make it virtually impossible to know whether a product lacks a disclosure. There are exceptions within exemptions that the average consumer can't possibly understand.

CRISPR-Cas9 has become immensely popular in recent years. George Church, a professor of genetics at Harvard Medical School notes that the technology is easy to use and is more than four times efficient than the previous best genome-editing tool. But it's not without its concerns. "I think the biggest limitation of CRISPR is it is not [one] hundred percent efficient," said Church. There is also the anomaly of "off-target effects," where DNA is cut at sites that can lead to the introduction of unintended mutations. Furthermore, Church noted that even when the system cuts are on target, there is always the chance of not getting a precise edit. He called this "genome vandalism." Traits could also unintentionally spread beyond the target population to other organisms through crossbreeding. Now *there's* a comforting thought.

"The pace of basic research discoveries has exploded, thanks to CRISPR," said biochemist Sam Sternberg, group leader of technology development at Berkeley, California-based Caribou Biosciences Inc., which is developing CRISPR-Cas9-based solutions for medicine, agriculture, and biological research. One example came in January 2018, when researchers announced that they may be able to stop fungi and other problems that threaten chocolate production using CRISPR-Cas9 to make the plants more resistant to disease. Confounding the new technologies, as with their predecessors in gene engineering, they must be required to fall in line with other related science, but have still managed a way to avoid being disclosed in product labeling.

What You Can Expect to See on Labeling

So, what do consumers have to look for? What do the new GMO labels look like? By January 1, 2022, you'll see three different labeling methods:

- Explicit text on food packaging, such as "Partially produced with genetic engineering"
- A symbol that represents bioengineering
- An electronic or digital link that can be scanned for more information

The law is limited to bioengineered foods intended for human consumption that contain more than five percent GMO ingredients. Instances where GMOs do not have to be labeled, include:

- Foods derived from animals, such as eggs, meat, and milk
- Refined ingredients such as oils and sugars
- Food served in a restaurant
- Foods manufactured and sold by very small merchants, such as local shops
- Non-food products

While the disclosure methods are confusing and burdensome, the exemptions allowed under the NBFDS are even worse, and are loaded with loopholes and contradictions. As a result, a mere fraction of products containing GMOs will actually end up being labeled. Animal feed, pet food, and personal care products are not affected at all. Only products that contain *detectable* GMO DNA will be labeled—which is a huge problem because many processed foods contain negligible amounts of beet sugar and canola oil at undetectable levels.

The Quiz

These exemptions make it virtually impossible to know whether a product lacks a disclosure because it is truly non-GMO or because it found a way to wiggle through one of the loopholes. There are exceptions within exemptions that the average consumer can't possibly understand. Don't believe it? Let's take a little quiz and look at a few examples of products. In each example, assume that all the **bolded ingredients** are derived from GMOs. The answers are inverted beneath each question.

Question #1
All of these soups contain GMOs, but only one will be labeled under the NBFDS. Can you tell which one?

1. Soup ingredients: **chicken** stock, **corn**, **chicken**, celery, carrots,
2. Soup ingredients: **chicken** stock, chicken, **corn**, celery, carrots,
3. Soup ingredients: vegetable broth (water, carrots, celery, paprika), chicken, **corn**, celery, carrots

Answer:
*In the list above, only the first example would be subject to disclosure. Multi-ingredient foods with meat as the first ingredient are exempt (except for seafood, rabbit, and venison) even when the animal consumed GMO feed. Water, stock, and broth don't count. This means the second example does not get a label because it has chicken as the second ingredient after stock, even though the very next ingredient is GMO corn. The third example does not get a label for the same reason even though it lists the non-exempt ingredients in the broth separately. **The first example gets a label** because it has corn as the second ingredient and chicken as the third.*

Question #2

All three of these frozen, breaded fish nuggets contain GMOs. Which one would get a BE label?

1. Fish product ingredients: minced catfish, water, **cornmeal, cornflour**, salt, **baking powder**, paprika, **canola oil, flavoring**
2. Fish product ingredients: minced pollock, wheat flour, water, **canola oil**, egg, **cornstarch**, onion powder, **flavoring**
3. Fish product ingredients: minced **chicken**, minced pollock, minced haddock, minced cod, enriched flour, **canola oil**, water, **yellow corn flour, sugar, yeast, natural flavor**

Answer:

In the list above, only the second example would be subject to disclosure. Products with seafood as the first ingredient are subject to labeling—except catfish, so the first example is exempt. The third example contains three types of seafood, which is subject to labeling, but it contains more chicken filler than it does pollock, so it is exempt too. Only the all-pollock fish nugget would be labeled—but only if the GMO DNA in the cornstarch or flavoring can be detected after processing.

Question #3

All of these chocolate candies contain GMOs. Can you tell which one would be labeled with a BE disclosure?

1. Chocolate bar ingredients: **sugar**, chocolate, cocoa butter, milk fat, **soy lecithin, canola oil, vanillin, artificial flavor**
2. Chocolate bar ingredients: **sugar**, cacao, cocoa butter, **soy lecithin, emulsifier, artificial flavor**
3. Chocolate bar ingredients: **sugar**, cocoa butter, whole milk powder, **soy lecithin**, natural vanilla

Answer:

It's impossible to tell for certain, but probably none of these. All three chocolates contain refined GMO ingredients. The sugar and canola oil can't be tested for GMOs; there is not enough intact DNA. The soy lecithin could possibly contain detectable GMO DNA in some circumstances, but not in others. The NBFDS only requires labeling if the GMO DNA is detectable in the finished product. Unfortunately, this policy just keeps consumers guessing.

Non-GMO Project©, used by permission[51]

Summary

As with the Nutrition Facts Panel that suddenly popped up on the sides of packages in 1994, government and science have finally begun to listen to consumers: They want to know what's in the food they eat and make educated decisions for themselves about whether or not they choose to buy the products.

Let's face it. Ever since being duped by big tobacco, consumers don't trust what they're being told by the government, lobbyists, and big companies. Although it's taken more than twenty-five years, consumers can finally read nutrition labels on fresh fruit and vegetables as well as the sides of packaging and determine for themselves how much fat, carbohydrate, sugars, protein, fiber, and salt they want in the products they consume.

In the next chapter, we'll delve into how to make sound choices, and how to use them to inform steps to reduce your risk for cancer by avoiding GMOs. Or, should I say, bioengineered food.

---

51 Can You Tell Which GMOs Will Be Labeled under the NBFDS?

CHAPTER SIX

Reducing the Burden of Cancer

GMO is a meaningless term. All the food we eat has been altered in some manner for over 10,000 years.
- Pamela Ronald

"You really should quit smoking."
"You should stay out of the sun or you'll get skin cancer."
"You should get that lump checked out."

How many times have you heard a friend or loved one getting read the riot act about the impending doom of succumbing to cancer? As they should. If caught in time, thirty to fifty percent of cancers can be prevented by using existing evidence-based prevention strategies, early detection of cancer, and patient management of those who develop cancer.

There are over 100 types of cancers throughout the world. In 2018, an estimated 1,735,350 new cases of cancer were diagnosed in the U.S. with 609,640 deaths from the disease.[52] More than thirty-eight percent of men and women will be diagnosed with cancer at some point during their lifetimes. The most common cancers are:

Breast cancer	Kidney and renal pelvis cancer
Lung and bronchus cancer	Endometrial cancer
Prostate cancer	Leukemia
Colon and rectum cancer	Pancreatic cancer
Melanoma of the skin	Thyroid cancer
Ovarian cancer	Liver cancer
NHL	Bladder cancer

The Diet Connection

Risk factors for all forms of cancer[53] include:

- Age
- Alcohol
- Cancer-causing substances
- Chronic inflammation
- Hormones
- Immunosuppression
- Infectious agents
- Obesity
- Radiation
- Sunlight
- Tobacco
- Diet

---

52 National Cancer Institute: Cancer Statistics - https://www.cancer.gov/about-cancer/understanding/statistics

53 Risk Factors for Cancer – National Cancer Institute - https://www.cancer.gov/about-cancer/causes-prevention/risk

But, wait. Did you say *diet*? What does diet have to do with getting cancer? As it turns out, a lot.

Since 1976, when GMOs hit the market, new evidence has surfaced about their role in causing or promoting numerous forms of cancer in humans and animals. Once thought to be the "Golden Boys" of twentieth-century agriculture practices, they've come under intense scrutiny. Consider these shocking statistics:

- After genetically modified soy hit the U.K. market, soy allergies increased by fifty percent
- When given a choice, cows, pigs, and rats, avoid eating GMO feed over non-GMO feed
- Reports from four U.K. villages revealed that twenty-five percent of the sheep died within a week after sheep herds grazed on Bt cotton plants.
- Workers at six villages succumbed to reactions of the skin, eyes, and upper respiratory tract after handling Bt cotton.
- In 2003, one hundred people living in the Philippines complained of skin, respiratory, and intestinal problems while the corn was shedding pollen after living next to a Bt cornfield.

Nevertheless, supporters of GMOs would have you believe those are only minor incidents, and that their advantages far outweigh their disadvantages. Supporters further claim that genetically modified plants grow faster than organic ones, are better for the environment, and produce more food for hungry populations. But are GMOs really as safe as we are led to believe? The truth is, GMOs are pathetic, unhealthy replacements for real food. More importantly, people have a right to know what they're eating and decide for themselves if they should buy these products.

Studies show that when DNA is altered it increases your risk of getting cancer.

It's no secret that legislation behind GMO labeling is woefully lagging behind consumers' demands. It wasn't until recently that congress was pressured into passing the National Bioengineered Food Disclosure Standard (NBFDS). The law requires the USDA to establish labeling standards for all genetically modified or bioengineered food. This standard allows people to make up their own minds whether to include GMOs in their diet, including foods that have been linked to cancer and covered up by the government, chemical companies, and large food producers. While the law was initially passed in 2016, it won't be "enforced" until January 1, 2022. In the meantime, consumers must take responsibility for educating themselves if they want to avoid buying GMO foods and products.

At the Center of the Debate

There's been a lot of hoo-haw over GMOs. Studies show that when DNA is altered it increases your risk of getting cancer. That's because the genetic substances in GMOs end up altering the DNA of humans and alter normal body functions. When this happens, a person is at risk for growing cancerous tumors. The cells are affected by this DNA modification and they end up functioning abnormally, which leads to cancer. The Washington D.C.-based Center for Food Safety[54], an anti-GMO organization, calls the genetic engineering of plants and animals

54 Center for Food Safety: https://www.centerforfoodsafety.org/

"one of the greatest and most intractable environmental challenges of the 21st century."

Recombinant bovine growth hormone (rBGH) is another manmade hormone marketed to dairy farmers to help increase milk production in cows. It has been used in the U.S. since the FDA approved its use in 1993.

As it turns out, milk produced from rBGH-treated cows contains more insulin-like growth factor 1 (IGF-1) than regular dairy products. IGF-1 represents one of the highest risk factors associated with breast and prostate cancer. Nearly every independent animal feeding safety study shows adverse or unexplained effects.

When genetically modified crops, such as corn or wheat, are used to create other foods, including corn tortillas or bread, there is a high probability that consuming these foods can cause an allergic reaction.

An allergy is a hypersensitive immune response that occurs when people come into contact with specific substances called allergens. Allergies can lead to red eyes, itchy rashes, swelling, runny noses, breathing difficulties, and can even prove fatal. Allergies are very common. Food-specific allergies affect 240-550 million people in the world. In the U.S., one out of every thirteen children suffers from food allergies, with the prevalence of childhood allergies increasing by more than fifty percent in the past twenty years.

The new labeling law makes it virtually impossible to interpret. There are exceptions to exceptions to exceptions. Even the experts don't completely understand how to employ them.

In one case[55], a pest-repelling protein used on corn to destroy insects in the field and only approved for animal feeding was cross-pollinated with unmodified crops and ultimately entered the human body. People with an allergy to the protein may be at risk for severe anaphylactic shock, and even death.

In late 2000, a California woman named Grace Booth went into anaphylactic shock after eating three tacos. After ruling out all other food allergies, she became suspicious about the corn in the tortillas she ate. Earlier that year, a consumer group found that some Taco Bell taco shells contain a pest-repelling protein called Cry9C. Originally from common soil bacteria, Cry9C used to destroy insect intestines, and was introduced into StarLink GMO corn to kill predatory caterpillars. The farmers weren't aware that StarLink corn had only been approved for animal feeding, and was never intended for human consumption because of concerns that Cry9C would be difficult to digest and cause an allergic reaction. However, it still entered the human food supply due to cross-pollination when the GMO corn was planted too close to unmodified crops, and the tortillas that Grace ate were soon recalled due to contamination from a GMO product.

On the flip side, Erma Levy, a research dietitian with Houston-based cancer-care giant MD Anderson claims, "To some degree, everything is genetically modified."

So what are savvy consumers to do? The new labeling law makes it virtually impossible to interpret. There are exceptions to exceptions to exceptions. Even the experts don't completely understand how to employ them. But fear not. There are simple steps you can take when reading GMO-labeled foods until the government and BigAg catch up...if they ever do. Here are a few beginning steps:

---

55 Harvard University: Nothing to Sneeze at: the Allergenicity of GMOs - http://sitn.hms.harvard.edu/flash/2015/allergies-and-gmos/

- **Know the most commonly modified crops.** Soybeans, corn, cotton, canola (for oil), squash, zucchini, and papaya are all popular GMOs used in a wide array of processed products. Whenever possible, choose alternatives to these GM crops[56].

Alfalfa	Pineapple
Apple	Plum
Argentine canola	Polish canola
Bean	Potato
Carnation	Rice
Chicory	Safflower
Cotton	Soybean
Cowpea	Squash
Eggplant	Sugar beet
Eucalyptus	Sugarcane
Flax	Sweet pepper
Maize	Tobacco
Melon	Tomato
Papaya	Wheat

- **Buy organic foods.** Organic foods are grown from non-GMO seeds. Look for the "organic" label on foods in the produce section.
- **Buy meat from grass-fed or pasture-fed animals.** Cows, chickens, pigs, and farmed fish are typically fed diets of genetically modified corn or alfalfa. Check that your meat is from animals that are grass-fed or pasture-fed.
- **Read the labels**[57]. The top two genetically modified crops are corn and soy. They're also the most widely

---

56 International Service for the Acquisition of Agriculture - http://www.isaaa.org/gmapprovaldatabase/cropslist/default.asp

57 MD Anderson Cancer Center: How to read a nutrition label - https://www.mdanderson.org/publications/focused-on-health/Howtoreadanutrtionlabel.h12-1590624.html

used ingredients. Avoid products that contain ingredients such as corn syrup and soy lecithin.

- **Buy brands labeled non-GM or GMO-free**[58]. Some products are labeled as non-GM or GMO-free, meaning that they do not use genetically modified ingredients. GMO-free food sources are listed on the Non-GMO Project website.
- **Shop at local farmers' markets or retailers**[59]. Most GM foods come from large industrial farms. Shop at local farmers' markets or sign up for a co-op.

You've probably heard the axiom, "shop the perimeter" of food stores. It's particularly important these days when just about everything we eat contains GMOs. Most highly processed foods lurk in the center isles of grocery stores. They're the Pop-Tarts, Cocoa Puffs, and Ritz Crackers mixed in with so-called "healthy foods."

Four crops are responsible for the majority of GMO foods: Corn, soy, canola, and sugar beets. Learning how to avoid the first three is simple, but sugar is harder. The main source of GMOs in our food supply is corn. The list of corn products is as long as your arm and, sometimes more mysterious. Dextrose, maltodextrin, and xanthan gum are all corn-based. Soy can pop up in unexpected places, including lecithin, an emulsifier.

Sugar is another thing altogether. It appears on product ingredient lists and is harder to pin down because, although almost all sugar beets are GMO, beet sugar represents a little

---

58 Verified Products - https://www.nongmoproject.org/find-non-gmo/verified-products/

59 Non-GMO Project - Verified Products - https://www.nongmoproject.org/find-non-gmo/verified-products/

less than half of the sugar we use in the U.S. Unless the label says "cane sugar," it's pretty much up for grabs.

If you bring your iPad into the store, after a couple of hours you can meticulously discover whether or not those Protein Bars, Pepperidge Farm Cookies, or Stouffer's frozen lasagna contain GM ingredients. Instead, learn the "first rule" of grocery shopping: If it's processed food, it probably contains GMOs.

If people really want to stop eating GMOs, it's relatively easy to do. By checking the ingredient lists, cutting way back on processed foods, and buying organic, you can rest assured you're making a non-GMO impact and reducing your risk for cancer. The problem is however, the percent of U.S. corn and soy used in genetically modified food is gradually increasing, meaning the food companies have us coming and going.

Unfortunately, it's going to take time before the government and big business are brought to their knees like their predecessors, Big Tobacco. In the meantime, it's going to have to be "every man for him (or her) self.

The Secrets to Buying Non-GMO

Animals, including chickens, cows, and pigs are typically fed from genetically modified feed such as corn. Ultimately, the GMO ends up finding its way into *you* through eating *their* meat. On the other hand, organic foods are safe because they're made from non-GMO seeds. Always read the labels when purchasing food, and go for foods that are labeled GMO-free. Always opt for animals you know are grass-fed, such as those raised in farms, and the same goes for dairy products.

To be honest, most people aren't even aware that they're eating GMO food. Nevertheless, they're entitled to know whether or not they are. Currently, there's no unifying principle about what does or does not go onto non-GMO labels, but people want to know what they're eating. They've learned over the years that eating trans-fats is not good for the heart and arteries, but that eating fiber is. Beverages loaded with sugar and caffeine are bad for the body, but fruit juices are good.

Since the inception of the Nutrition Facts Panel in 1994[60], labeling tells you what you're eating, and country-of-origin labels allow you to make sound decisions based on ideals you have about domestic and foreign foods. Unfortunately, it's going to take time before the government and big business are brought to their knees in the same way as their predecessors, Big Tobacco. In the meantime, it's going to have to be "every man for him (or her) self."

Summary

Until consumers learn how to ramp up to the confusing tactics used by big food producers, remember these four important steps[61] to reduce your risk for cancer and other diseases caused by GMO foods:

---

60 Food Dive - The origins and evolution of Nutrition Facts labeling - https://www.fooddive.com/news/the-origins-and-evolution-of-nutrition-facts-labeling/507016/#:~:text=Consequently%2C%20the%20U.S.%20became%20the%20first%20country%20to,Gould%20Net%20Weight%20Amendment%20to%20the%201906%20Act.

61 The Real Risks of GMO Foods & How to Avoid - https://draxe.com/nutrition/the-real-risks-of-gmo-foods-how-to-avoid/

1. **Buy Certified Organic:** Products can be one hundred percent organic or they can be "made with organic ingredients." Items "made with organic ingredients" must contain at least seventy percent organic ingredients, but one hundred percent of those ingredients still must be non-GMO.

2. **Choose Items with Certified Non-GMO Labels:** Look for labeling such as the Non-GMO Project seal on packaging to ensure the product is Non-GMO Project Verified.

3. **Shop Local:** Shop at small local farms can also help to reduce your likelihood of buying and consuming GMOs. Talk to the farmers at your local farmers' markets, visit the farms yourself and get to know the non-GMO options in your own backyard.

4. **Read Labels Carefully:** Read labels carefully, especially on items such as snack foods, to avoid common genetically engineered ingredients. The Center for Food Safety[62] has a very helpful list of the most common genetically engineered "Big Five" ingredients commonly found in processed foods:

   - **Corn:** Corn flour/meal/oil/starch/gluten/syrup, and sweeteners such as fructose, dextrose, and glucose
   - **Beet Sugar:** Sugar that's not specified as one hundred percent cane sugar is likely from GE sugar beets
   - **Soy:** Soy flour, lecithin, protein, isolate, and isoflavone as well as soy-derived vegetable oil and vegetable protein
   - **Canola:** Canola oil (also called rapeseed oil)
   - **Cotton:** Cottonseed oil

---

62 Tips for Avoiding GMOs - https://www.centerforfoodsafety.org/issues/311/ge-foods/shoppers-guide-to-avoiding-ge-food/1846/tips-for-avoiding-gmos

CHAPTER SEVEN

Conclusions

W e've been domesticating plants and animals for more than 12,000 years, mostly through selective and artificial breeding when farmers began dinking around with crops and livestock because they were desperate to eke out a bit more food from their minuscule plots of land. They were more or less successful until big business and greed got into the mix. To this day, they're at the center of one of the most hotly contested debates in modern science, with as many opponents as supporters. Why? It's simple: People want to know what they're eating and if it's safe for their families.

Unknown dangers lurk deep within ears of corn, tomatoes, and other popular foods—foods that should be labeled and safely controlled, allowing consumers to decide for themselves whether or not they're going to pass on that box of Pop-Tarts for a handful of organic carrots.

Making matters worse is federally-mandated product labeling, using a convoluted maze of rules, requirements, and regulations that would give Alice in Wonderland a migraine headache.

At the heart of the controversy are systems of convoluted cover-ups, accompanied by out-and-out fraud by big biotech companies such Bayer, B.A.SF, Dow AgroScience, Dupont Pioneer, Monsanto, and Syngenta. They were (and still are) the golden boys behind the squabbles over GMOs that are currently gripping our country.

The chief threat is Monsanto, who famously manufactured Agent Orange between 1961 and 1971 and was responsible for more than 400,000 deaths and injuries of American soldiers and four million Vietnamese after deforesting Vietnam, Cambodia, and Laos during the Vietnam conflict. Since then, they've leaped into big agriculture by producing Roundup® —a powerful herbicide designed to repel weeds, insects, and other threats to crops. While it is an effective weed killer and pesticide, it's also one of the most lethal substances known to man. Monsanto is doing its best to promote a double-edged sword: Increasing GMOs while hiding them from consumers.

Today, genetically modified alfalfa, apples, canola, corn, cotton, eggplant, papaya, pink flesh pineapple, potatoes, salmon, soybeans, sugar beets, and summer squash make millions for agricultural giants, farmers, and food producers. At the same time, consumers resist the idea of eating "counterfeit" or Frankenfood that's misrepresented as something that's good for them. There's something inherently deceptive about having it snuck onto supermarket shelves and presented as real food.

Since the early 1990s, genetically modified foods have been approved for use in more than seventy percent of all processed foods in domestic supermarkets, from pizza, potato chips, cookies, ice cream, salad dressing, corn syrup, to baking powder—all contain ingredients from bio-engineered soybeans, corn, or canola plants. Chances are, if you have food in your pantry, you're eating bioengineered food.

Despite support from pro-labeling consumer groups, the first disclosure requirement for documenting ingredients in GMOs didn't take effect until January 1, 2020, even though compliance won't actually be enforceable until January 1, 2022. In the meantime, government, lobbying firms, and big food producers are scurrying around, looking for more deceptive ways to sneak their existing products under the wire without destroying the profitable models they already have in place. Making matters worse is federally-mandated product labeling, using a convoluted maze of rules, requirements, and regulations that would give Alice in Wonderland a migraine headache.

Roundup Ready® Gets into the Market

To date, American food producers have applied more than 1.8 million tons of glyphosate-herbicides since its introduction. Worldwide, more than 9.4 million tons of the chemical has been sprayed on fields; enough to shower half a pound of Roundup® on every cultivated acre of land in the world. Glyphosate use has risen fifteen-fold since Roundup Ready® GMO crops were first introduced.

In 2015, the World Health Organization's International Agency for Research on Cancer (IARC) classified glyphosate as "probably carcinogenic to humans[63]" after reviewing years of published and peer-reviewed scientific studies. The EPA's Cancer Assessment Review Committee (CARC) issued a report in September of 2016, concluding that glyphosate was "not likely to be carcinogenic to humans" at doses relevant to human health

At the same time, the EPA's Office of Research and Development claimed that EPA's Office of Pesticide Programs had not followed proper protocols in its evaluation of glyphosate, and said that the resulting evidence could be deemed to support a likely carcinogenic or suggestive evidence of carcinogenicity classification. It appears that even the same government office can't agree on the carcinogenic threat of agricultural herbicides.

As recent as April 2019, when the EPA reaffirmed its position that glyphosate poses no risk to public health, the U.S. Agency for Toxic Substances and Disease Registry (ATSDR) reported links between glyphosate and cancer. If your head isn't spinning by now, it should be. How on earth are consumers supposed to arrive at meaningful conclusions when even the U.S. government can't?

Chances are, your children—even those who are just beginning their lives in utero—are already exposed to hundreds of toxins, with the threat of cancer around every turn.

---

63 IARC Monographs Volume 112: evaluation of five organophosphate insecticides and herbicide - https://www.iarc.fr/wp-content/uploads/2018/07/MonographVolume112-1.pdf

Since glyphosate products were introduced into the market, more than 42,000 people have filed lawsuits against Monsanto Company claiming that exposure to its Roundup® herbicide caused them or their loved ones to develop NHL, and that Monsanto covered up known risks. While the backgrounds of the lawsuits vary, one thing that all of them have in common is the validated plaintiff's claim that Roundup® was a defective product and unreasonably dangerous to consumers, and Monsanto knew or should have known that glyphosate caused cancer and other illnesses, and failed to properly warn consumers of the risks.

Data from a USDA 2016 study showed detectable pesticide levels in eighty-five percent of more than 10,000 foods sampled—everything from mushrooms to grapes and green beans. At the same time, the government claims there are little to no health risks to consumers. But, with so much money and influence on the line, they're not likely to turn a blind eye and admit the truth.

Does all this sound familiar? If you're one of the thousands of people who got hooked on cigarettes by big tobacco back in the 1950s and 1960s, you know that big business and the government can't be trusted to tell consumers the truth; the very consumers who keep them in business and make them rich.

If you've eaten commercially processed foods, your DNA could already be damaged from years of eating so-called "whole foods" that are "low-fat," "gluten-free," and every other fad touted by the media. Your children—even those who are just beginning their lives in utero—could already be exposed to hundreds of toxins, with the threat of cancer around every turn.

Major health groups, including the American Medical Association and World Health Organization who we've come to respect and turn to for valid, authentic information, have concluded from their research of independent groups world-wide that genetically modified foods are "safe for consumers, free of threats to organ health, mutations, pregnancy, and off-spring." Consumer advocates with "no dogs in the race" suggest otherwise—compelling reasons why we shouldn't trust the government and big business. They're simply in it for the money.

Although scientists claim that they've been able to manipulate data indicating that GMOs are not toxic to the animals that eat them, they've failed to support long-term studies in humans for one reason: Studies to back up human safety are nowhere to be found. One of the only valid studies to come close was published in November 2012, in the *Journal of Food and Chemical Toxicology*, by researchers at France's Caen University. They discovered hormonal and sex-related problems in females that included mammary tumors, pituitary, and kidney problems, while males died mostly from kidney failure. Up to fifty percent of the male rats and seventy percent of females died prematurely, compared with only thirty and twenty percent in the control group, respectively.

How can this be possible? How can consumers be told GMO foods are safe for consumption? Because government and big business like things exactly the way they are, making money hand over fist with little or no concern for the health of consumers. They've found ways to manipulate the data consumers are fed. Just the way big tobacco did back in the 1950s.

Organic Food Enters the Market

Years ago, the founders of giant chain grocery stores were concerned that consumers were being duped by large-scale growers trying to muscle their way into the popularity of organic food sales. Their solution was the first set of standards identifying organic food packaging. But it wasn't until 1973, when Oregon became the first state to pass a law regulating organic food production. After several failed attempts, a law establishing the USDA organic standards went into effect in February 2001. Since then, large-scale commercial farmers hit the ground running by cutting corners, misinterpreting, and bending the law to their benefit as they tried to take advantage of lax USDA enforcement.

As the organic food production industry matures and becomes more popular with consumers, organic farmers and food producers face stiff competition from large companies that primarily produce conventional food, yet want to slither in through the back door with "organic" products, eschewing formal guidelines. So, it's up to consumers to do their homework.

If organic food is so popular with consumers, why doesn't the government and BigAg get busy growing more? Because the demand for organic product sales vastly outstrips the supply, sometimes leading to outright fraud. In China—one of the biggest soybean exporters to the U.S.—farmers have enough trouble following their own laws, let alone U.S. organic rules, which pretty much sums up the current state of food and drug enforcement.

Opposition to genetically modified organisms is fierce. One of the most visible groups is the Non-GMO Project. It states, "Most developed nations do not consider GMOs to be safe. In more than sixty countries around the world, including Australia, Japan, and all of the countries in the European Union, there are significant restrictions or outright bans on the production and sale of GMOs." Opponents of genetically modified foods claim that scientists are "playing God" with the products we consume.

To make matters worse, consumers and federal regulators can't seem to agree on exactly what should or shouldn't be included in product labeling. They run the gamut from the country of origin to ingredients that pose risk to some people like peanuts and gluten, as well as others like salt that most health authorities agree we should all limit. However, most do agree that consumers have a right to know whether or not the products they buy are grown using herbicide-intensive agriculture. At the same time, the American Medical Association and the American Association for the Advancement of Science take the position that absent scientific evidence of harm, even voluntary labeling is misleading and will falsely alarm consumers.

Labeling of GMO products in the U.S. and Canada is voluntary, while countries in the European Union mandate that all food—including processed food or animal feed containing just under one percent and higher of approved GMOs—must be labeled. The result has led to international trade disputes, litigation, and protests. Experience has shown that clear, simple GMO labeling helps to assuage questions and confusion by consumers.

The problem is, there are plenty of opportunities for scurrilous companies opposed to transparent labeling practices to bury information, without confirming their products contain GMOs or ingredients made from them. Instead of requiring a simple symbol or text disclosure, the new USDA rule allows companies to get away with workarounds such as QR codes, hyperlinks, and toll-free phone numbers to cloud their use of genetic engineering—all of which make it impossible for consumers standing in the produce department, holding a bunch of radishes in one hand, with a bag of Doritos in the other, wondering to themselves, "Which of these should I buy?"

So, what do consumers have to look forward to? What do the new GMO labels look like? No later than January 1, 2022, you'll see three different labeling methods:

- Explicit text on food packaging, such as "Partially produced with genetic engineering"
- A symbol that represents bioengineering
- An electronic or digital link that can be scanned for more information

The law is limited to bioengineered foods intended for human consumption that contain more than five percent GMO ingredients. Instances, where GMOs do not have to be labeled include:

- Foods derived from animals, such as eggs, meat, and milk
- Refined ingredients, including oils and sugars
- Food served in a restaurant
- Foods manufactured and sold by very small merchants such as local shops
- Non-food products

While the disclosure methods are confusing and burdensome, the exemptions allowed are even worse, and are loaded with loopholes and contradictions. As a result, a mere fraction of products containing GMOs will actually end up being labeled.

Let's face it. Ever since being duped by big tobacco, consumers simply don't trust what they're told by the government, lobbying, and industry giants. Although it's taken more than twenty-five years, consumers can finally read nutrition labels on fresh fruit and vegetables as well as the sides of packaging and determine for themselves how much fat, carbohydrate, sugars, protein, fiber, and salt they want to consume in the products they buy.

GMOs and the Threat of Cancer

When genetically modified organisms hit the market in 1976, new evidence surfaced about their role in causing or promoting numerous forms of cancer in humans and animals. That's because the genetic substances in GMOs end up altering the DNA of humans, and also alter normal body functions. When this happens, a person is at risk for growing cancerous tumors.

The new labeling law is impossible to interpret. There are exceptions to exceptions to exceptions. Even the experts don't completely understand how to deal with them. But fear not. There are simple steps consumers can take when reading GMO-labeled foods until the government and BigAg catch up. First, identify the most commonly modified crops; second, whenever possible, buy organic foods; third, buy meat from grass-fed or pasture-fed animals; next, always read the labels; next, buy brands labeled non-GM or GMO-free, and finally, shop at local farmers' markets or retailers.

The reality is, most of the public couldn't care less about GMOs. When you ask them GMO-specific questions such as, "Do you think genetically engineered foods should have labels?" they are likely to say "yes" because it sounds like a good thing to do.

If you really want to stop eating GMOs, it's relatively easy to do. By checking ingredient lists, eliminating processed foods, and buying organic, you can rest assured you're making a non-GMO impact and reducing your risk for cancer. The problem is, the percentage of U.S. corn and soy used in genetically modified food is gradually increasing, meaning the food companies have us coming and going.

Most people aren't aware that they're eating GMO food. Currently, there's no unifying principle about what does or does not go onto non-GMO labels. But people still want to believe that they know what they're eating.

The reality is, most of the public couldn't care less about GMOs. When you ask them GMO-specific questions like, "Do you think genetically engineered foods should have labels?" they are likely to say "yes" because it sounds like the right thing to do. After all, who wouldn't want genetically modified food labeled? But when you ask them an open-ended question like, "What specific information would you like to see on food labels that is not already there?" fewer than seven percent mention GMOs. Barely twenty-five percent believe they've eaten genetically modified food in the past. Only forty-five percent think GMOs are safe to eat. Given that probably all of us have eaten GMOs, and the scientific community seems to agree they are safe to eat, failing any long-term human studies being conducted, no one definitively knows.

Labeling issues are chewing up valuable resources that could be better spent on advancing science. Millions of dollars are wasted that could be used for GMO labeling food products. Legislative efforts, at both the state and federal level on both sides of the equation, are being funded by people who care deeply about our food and how it's regulated. Given the big companies' access to power, those activists are an important check, and their efforts are a critical resource.

Scott Faber, executive director of Washington D.C.-based Just Label It, says, "There are many pressing, equally important food supply issues: that our food is safe, that people have enough to eat, that we grow our food in ways that protect the environment, that we raise animals humanely, that we treat workers with dignity, and that people have the ability to make choices." He goes on to say, "Smart companies are recognizing that the long-term trend is toward more disclosure and not less." That may be the single best argument for GMO labeling. Like big tobacco experienced, transparency should be the first way companies compete.

According to Monsanto, its efforts are steeped in altruistic actions. The company claims it wants to help impoverished nations by giving them GMOs. But that's debatable. Money and power fuels deception. The business model behind Monsanto is to eliminate the competition by stealing people's land. Patents on seeds and converting them to GMOs make it possible for biotech companies like Monsanto to take over the entire agriculture industry.

Monsanto is one of the most corrupt companies on the planet. They begin the process by getting the farmer to sign their technology agreement. The agreement allows Monsanto to:

- Conduct property investigations
- Expose the farmer to enormous financial liability
- Bind the farmer to Monsanto's oversight for multiple years
- Prevent farmers from selling or reusing their seeds

It can sue farmers for patent infringement if they try to reuse their seeds. In the past, farmers who planted their saved seeds faced severe financial penalties. Many went bankrupt. The practice has ruined the economy of Indian cotton farmers—innocent farmers who had to take out massive loans to buy the seeds and their weed killers. When the GMO crops failed, the farmers failed to repay their loans, often resulting in farmers in India committing suicide[64] at an alarming rate.

One thing is certain: Until big businesses get out of bed with the government, honest communication with consumers simply won't happen. There is no impetus to discover and label toxic products when they currently represent millions of dollars in revenue for BigAg companies, lobbyists, and the government. But there are things consumers can do: They can support legislation with their pocketbooks. Money talks. When wholesale grocers begin to experience the impact of negative sales due to improper labeling practices, you can bet they'll use their collective pressure to make things right. Until that happens, the best method is to protect yourself. Get educated, read the labels, and buy organic food.

Would knowing which foods pose fewer threats from cancer have saved my mom? That's a good question; one I'll never know. But at least she would have known which foods she was or wasn't eating were exacerbating her condition. That's a start.

---

64 Over 12,000 farmer suicides per year, Centre tells Supreme Court - https://timesofindia.indiatimes.com/india/over-12000-farmer-suicides-per-year-centre-tells-supreme-court/article-show/58486441.cms

REFERENCES

1. What's a GMO? Are GMOs Safe? Learn the Shocking Truth - https://youtu.be/87p49NLeI_s
2. Cancer, Sugar & GMOs - https://youtu.be/UoKvZSs8lxs
3. Top 20 GMO Foods and Ingredients to Avoid - https://globalhealing.com/natural-health/top-20-gmo-foods-and-ingredients-to-avoid/
4. Neil deGrasse Tyson gets to the bottom of GMOs - https://youtu.be/aMDhUsxom0U
5. Crops , wheat, soybeans, corn and vegetables - https://gmoanswers.com/gmos-in-the-us?gclid=Cj0KCQjw-g8n5BRCdARIsALxKb95827VI3LS2UXPx7t-190s0r-BrEP0q9b0BwjYcauBPnmzqKDgOD9ycaAnumEALw_wcB
6. What does Organic mean - https://www.mashed.com/176421/what-does-organic-food-really-mean/
7. Info1 - https://www.collective-evolution.com/2018/02/09/hundreds-of-scientists-tell-the-world-that-the-gmo-cancer-link-is-real/
8. "Peer Reviewed:" Science Losing Credibility As Large Amounts Of Research Shown To Be False
9. RETRACTED: Long term toxicity of a Roundup herbicide and a Roundup-tolerant genetically modified maize
10. How Monsanto Genetically Modifies Our Food Compared To What Happens Naturally In Nature

11. Study of complete RNA collection of fruit fly uncovers unprecedented complexity - https://archive.news.indiana.edu/releases/iu/2014/03/drosophila-transcriptome-diversity-uncovered.shtml

12. World Health Organization Says Processed Meat Causes Cancer - https://amp.cancer.org/latest-news/world-health-organization-says-processed-meat-causes-cancer.html

13. The Link Between Processed Foods and Cancer - https://www.lifespan.org/lifespan-living/link-between-processed-foods-and-cancer

14. Study suggests possible link between highly processed foods and cancer - https://www.bmj.com/company/newsroom/study-suggests-possible-link-between-highly-processed-foods-and-cancer/

15. What does organic food really mean? - https://www.mashed.com/176421/what-does-organic-food-really-mean/

16. National List of Allowed and Prohibited Substances - https://www.ecfr.gov/cgi-bin/text-idx?c=ecfr&SID=9874504b6f1025eb0e6b67cadf9d3b40&rgn=div6&view=text&node=7:3.1.1.9.32.7&idno=7#sg7.3.205.g.sg0

17. Higher PUFA and n-3 PUFA, conjugated linoleic acid, α-tocopherol and iron, but lower iodine and selenium concentrations in organic milk: a systematic literature review and meta- and redundancy analyses - https://www.cambridge.org/core/journals/british-journal-of-nutrition/article/div-classtitlehigher-pufa-and-span-classitalicnspan-3-pufa-conjugated-linoleic-acid-span-classitalicspan-tocopherol-and-iron-but-lower-iodine-and-selenium-concentrations-in-organic-milk-a-systematic-liter-

ature-review-and-meta-and-redundancy-analysesdiv/
A7587A524F4235D8E98423E1F73B6C05

18. Organic Production & Handling Standards - https://
www.ams.usda.gov/publications/content/
organic-production-handling-standards

19. CDC study attempts to assess outbreak risk from
organic food - https://www.foodsafetynews.
com/2016/11/cdc-study-attempts-to-assess-out-
break-risk-from-organic-food/#.WsY9eS7waUl

20. Why GMOs Don't Cause Cancer - https://www.
forbes.com/sites/gmoanswers/2016/06/01/
why-gmos-dont-cause-cancer/#404583306bc8

21. GMO labeling: Is the fight worth it? - https://www.
washingtonpost.com/lifestyle/food/gmo-labeling-is-
the-fight-worth-it/2014/01/13/f7fa1352-7728-11e3-
b1c5-739e63e9c9a7_story.html?tid=a_inl_manual

22. GMO Labeling Isn't Dead: See Which States Are Leading the Fight - http://www.justlabelit.org/press-cen-
ter/press-items/gmo-labeling-isnt-dead-see-which-
states-are-leading-the-fight/

23. California Proposition 37, Mandatory Labeling of Genetically Engineered Food (2012) - https://ballotpe-
dia.org/California_Proposition_37,_Mandatory_La-
beling_of_Genetically_Engineered_Food_(2012)

24. US requires labeling of GMO foods as "bioengineered" - https://cen.acs.org/policy/regulation/
US-requires-labeling-GMO-foods/96/web/2018/12

25. Biotechnology Innovation Organization - https://
www.bio.org/

26. GMO Facts

27. What Are GMOs and GM Foods?

28. GMO Answers - https://gmoanswers.com/

29. National Bioengineered Food Disclosure Standard - https://www.federalregister.gov/documents/2018/12/21/2018-27283/national-bioengineered-food-disclosure-standard

30. Encyclopedia Britannica: Rudolf Jaenisch - https://www.britannica.com/biography/Rudolf-Jaenisch

31. Genetically modified foods in China and the United States: A primer of regulation and intellectual property protection - https://www.sciencedirect.com/science/article/pii/S2213453016300076

32. Food Science and Food Biotechnology - https://bit.ly/3hcFgRS

33. Genetically Engineered Crops in the United States - https://www.ers.usda.gov/webdocs/publications/45179/43668_err162.pdf

34. GMO crops have been increasing yield for 20 years, with more progress ahead - https://allianceforscience.cornell.edu/blog/2018/02/gmo-crops-increasing-yield-20-years-progress-ahead/

35. The Superpowers of Genetically Modified Pigs - https://www.the-scientist.com/notebook/the-superpowers-of-genetically-modified-pigs-64513

36. Convention on Biological Diversity: About the Protocol - http://bch.cbd.int/protocol/background/

37. Worlds Apart? The Reception of Genetically Modified Foods in Europe and the U.S. - https://science.sciencemag.org/content/285/5426/384

38. American Medical Association: REPORT 2 OF THE COUNCIL ON SCIENCE AND PUBLIC HEALTH (A-12) Labeling of Bioengineered Foods - https://web.archive.org/web/20120907023039/http:/www.ama-assn.org/resources/doc/csaph/a12-csaph2-bioengineeredfoods.pdf

39. Critical Reviews in Biotechnology: An overview of the last 10 years of genetically engineered crop safety research - https://www.pps.net/cms/lib/OR01913224/Centricity/Domain/3337/peer%20reviewed%20meta%20study%20on%20GMOs%20copy.pdf

40. Playing God? Synthetic biology as a theological and ethical challenge - https://www.ncbi.nlm.nih.gov/pmc/articles/PMC2759421/

41. Complementary Medicine, Refusal of Conventional Cancer Therapy, and Survival Among Patients With Curable Cancers - https://jamanetwork.com/journals/jamaoncology/article-abstract/2687972

42. Natural Cancer 'Cures': What Are the Risks? - https://www.yalemedicine.org/stories/natural-cancer-therapy-risks/

43. GMOs, Profits Over Health Is Monsanto's Business Model - https://sunshinefoodandvitamin.com/gmos-profit-over-health/

44. A Brief Explanation about GMOs Companies - https://www.tiredearth.com/articles/brief-explanation-about-gmos-companies

45. A new rule requires GMO products to be labeled by 2022, and some food companies are rejoicing - https://www.businessinsider.com/gmo-products-must-be-labeled-by-2022-usda-2018-12

46. Can You Tell Which GMOs Will Be Labeled under the NBFDS? - https://livingnongmo.org/2019/01/09/can-you-tell-which-gmos-will-be-labeled-under-the-nbfds/

47. Are GMOs the key to global food security? - https://www.devex.com/news/are-gmos-the-key-to-global-food-security-91862

48. Here's The Real Reason Why GMOs Are Bad, And Why They May Save Humanity - https://www.forbes.com/sites/erikkobayashisolomon/2019/02/15/heres-the-real-reason-why-gmos-are-bad-and-why-they-may-save-humanity/#4cc460844877

49. GMO Labeling - https://ota.com/advocacy/gmos/gmo-labeling

50. Everything you need to know about GMO labeling in 2020 –

51. Everything you need to know about GMO labeling in 2020 - https://www.watchusgrow.org/2019/01/08/everything-you-need-to-know-about-gmo-labeling-in-2019/

52. Why We Need Mandatory Labeling of GMO Products - https://www.statnews.com/2020/02/19/why-we-need-mandatory-labeling-of-gmo-products/

53. Americans Deserve Better than the USDA's GMO Labeling Law - https://livingnongmo.org/2019/01/04/americans-deserve-better-than-the-usdas-gmo-labeling-law/

54. Can You Tell Which GMOs Will Be Labeled under the NBFDS? - https://livingnongmo.org/2019/01/09/can-you-tell-which-gmos-will-be-labeled-under-the-nbfds/

55. Little evidence of health benefits from organic foods, study finds - https://med.stanford.edu/news/all-news/2012/09/little-evidence-of-health-benefits-from-organic-foods-study-finds.html

56. Aspartame: Decades of Science Point to Serious Health Risks - https://usrtk.org/sweeteners/aspartame_health_risks/

57.   Ballotpedia - https://ballotpedia.org/California_Prop-
       osition_37,_Mandatory_Labeling_of_Genetically_En-
       gineered_Food_(2012)

58.   What Is the Definition of Organic Food? - https://
       www.medicinenet.com/what_is_the_definition_of_
       organic_food/views.htm

59.   Organic Foods Guide: When To Buy (or Not Buy)
       Organic - https://www.medicinenet.com/organic_
       foods_pictures_slideshow/article.htm

60.   Organic 101: What the USDA Organic Label Means
       - https://www.usda.gov/media/blog/2012/03/22/
       organic-101-what-usda-organic-label-means

61.   Organic 101: What Organic Farming (and Process-
       ing) Doesn't Allow - https://www.usda.gov/media/
       blog/2011/12/16/organic-101-what-organic-farm-
       ing-and-processing-doesnt-allow

62.   Organic Foods: What You Need to Know - https://
       www.helpguide.org/articles/healthy-eating/organic-
       foods.htm

63.   National Cancer Institute - https://www.cancer.gov/
       about-cancer/causes-prevention/risk

64.   Do GMOs cause cancer? - https://www.mdanderson.
       org/publications/focused-on-health/gmos-cancer.
       h15-1589046.html

65.   Is There Evidence That GMOs Can Cause Cancer?
       - https://blog.dana-farber.org/insight/2019/08/
       is-there-evidence-that-gmos-can-cause-cancer/

66.   GMO and Link to Cancer - https://www.awaremed.
       com/dr-dalal-akoury/cancer-risk-gmo-link-cancer/

67.   Why GMOs Are No Friend To Cancer Patients - https://
       www.cancerwisdom.net/gmo-health-risks/

ABOUT THE AUTHOR

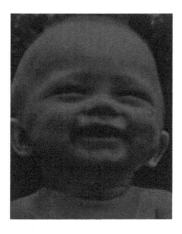

Elliot Steinberg is an independent businessman, who lives in Southern California with his wife and children. He studied medicine and finance and worked for the largest food corporation in the world. It was around this time that Mr. Steinberg discovered that there are secrets that both the major food industry and government do not want the public to know about. For the past ten years, Mr. Steinberg has become a devout supporter of food labeling. He has also held seminars and public speeches about the dangers of GMO's and their irrefutable connection to cancer and other life-threatening diseases. Mr. Steinberg has been an active Greenpeace member since the early 1980's and continues to serve as a voice for the consumer.

Made in the USA
Coppell, TX
05 January 2022

70519295R10079